Nature Immersion for Postpartum Healing

A Guided Journey to Exercise,
Mental Wellness & Emotional Balance

Postpartum Doula
Nature Immersion Guide
Ghene`t Lee-Yong

Nature Immersion for Postpartum Healing

A Guided Journey to Exercise, Mental Wellness & Emotional Balance

Copyright © 2025. Ghene`t Lee-Yong

All rights reserved. No part of this publication may be reproduced, distributed, or transmitted in any form or by any means, including photocopying, recording, or other electronic or mechanical methods, without the prior written permission of the publisher, except in the case of brief quotations embodied in critical reviews and certain other noncommercial uses permitted by copyright law. For permission requests, write to the publisher, addressed "Attention: Permissions Coordinator," at the address below.

ghenetleeyong@gmail.com

ISBN: 979-8-9935722-0-8

Book Design by Transcendent Publishing

No part of this work is to be used to train AI of any form.

This workbook is not intended as a substitute for the medical advice of a medical professional. The reader is advised to regularly consult with a physician on matters relating to his/her health (physical and mental) and particularly with respect to any symptoms that may require medical attention. Always consult your medical health physician when starting new exercise activities. Always consult with your medical health physician when starting or introducing new foods, herbs, or ingredients to your daily diet.

TABLE OF CONTENTS

Introduction..v

Section I: Emotional Wellness and Mental Health.............1
Chapter 1: Understanding Postpartum Emotional Changes 3
Chapter 2: Building Your Support Network...................9
Chapter 3: Recognizing Your Evolving Identity 17
Chapter 4: Mindfulness and Mental Hygiene for New Parents....25
Chapter 5: Journaling for Emotional Clarity 33
Chapter 6: Seeking Professional Support When Needed.........43
Nature Immersion: Step One - Observe 47

Section II: Physical Recovery and Self-Care 59
Chapter 7: The Fourth Trimester: A Look at Traditional and Cultural Practices Around Hygiene 61
Chapter 8: Healing After Birth: Natural Remedies and Tips......67
Chapter 9: Gentle Movement and Stretching for Recovery.......75
Chapter 10: Rest, Sleep, and Nutrition......................81
Chapter 11: Creating a Healthy Home Environment 85
Nature Immersion: Step Two - Connect....................91

Section III: Navigating Relationships 101
Chapter 12: There is Love Enough for All 103
Nature Immersion: Step Three - Accept 115

Section IV: Practical Parenting Tips 123
Chapter 13: Newborn Care 125
Chapter 14: Balancing Responsibilities and Self-Care.........133
Nature Immersion: Step Four – Engage 139

Section V: Finding Joy in the Postpartum Period 147
Chapter 15: Nature Immersion for Postpartum Healing........149
Chapter 16: Embracing Imperfection: Letting Go of
"Perfect Parenting" 153
Chapter 17: Fun, Simple Activities to Enjoy with Your Baby 157
Nature Immersion: Step Five - Solitude 163

Section VI: Honoring Fathers and Partners on the
Postpartum Path..171
Chapter 18: The Invisible Struggle: Fatherhood and Mental
Health After Birth 173
Chapter 19: Showing Up with Love: Everyday Ways to Support
and Stay Connected 177
Nature Immersion: Step Six - I AM 183
Bonus Journal Reflection 191
Nature as Your Guide: Walking Into Your Next Season........193
Acknowledgments 195
Appendix I: Recipes 197
Bibliography..211
About the Author..215

INTRODUCTION

Hello!

My name is Ghene`t (Janae), and I am a mother of two, a certified Postpartum Doula, and an Early Childhood Educator with over two decades of experience. My journey in early childhood education began when I was still a teenager, drawn to the joy of nurturing children and supporting families through their most tender seasons. Since then, I have led parenting workshops, earned a bachelor's degree in Cognitive Development across the lifespan (birth to geriatric), and created social media content focused on empowering families from the newborn stage and beyond.

My calling as a postpartum doula began when my son was two years old. I recognized how deeply families need compassionate, holistic support during the postpartum transition. Over time, I also noticed a growing disconnect between children, parents, and the natural world—a gap I felt compelled to address. As both an educator and a mother, I've seen firsthand how nature immersion supports emotional regulation, cognitive growth, and family bonding. Through this book, I aim to provide practical tools and heartfelt encouragement to help families reconnect with nature as a healing and developmental resource throughout their parenting journey.

Nine months of pregnancy, nine months of preparation, nine months of planning and anticipation—and now, the moment has finally come and gone.

Postpartum recovery is so much more than doctor's visits and monitoring your vitals. It involves all of you—your emotions, your sense of self, your shifting hormones, and the deep transformation that comes with motherhood. A holistic approach to healing the first forty days and beyond ensures that every aspect of recovery is supported.

This book is designed to inspire and guide you toward incorporating nature immersion into your weekly routine. It offers bite-sized portions of information because I know you are busy with the demanding and beautiful work of caring for your little one. These insights will encourage you to step outside, engage with nature, move your body, and nurture your mental well-being.

One of the greatest gifts of nature immersion as a parent is the opportunity to reconnect with your childlike wonder. You get to pick up sticks, marvel at rocks, and delight in the simple beauty of the natural world. You get to see the world with curiosity and openness. In nature, we find ourselves—because we, too, are nature. We are natural beings!

Nature immersion provides a gentle, holistic approach to postpartum recovery, supporting not just the body but also the mind and spirit.

A Special Note: When I speak of nature immersion, connection, mindfulness, or meditation, I am not referring to any specific religious practice. These concepts are simply ways to cultivate self-awareness and presence, to ease into movement, and to foster a deeper sense of connection and belonging to the world around us. Any mention of spirituality is not intended as religious guidance or to conflict with your personal beliefs. Instead, it reflects the inner self, identity, and knowingness that we often neglect in the midst of motherhood.

With that said, I invite you to embrace this journey. Enjoy your nature-immersion experience!

Matrescence

Embracing motherhood is a transformative journey that brings with it profound emotional shifts. Understanding and nurturing your emotional well-being during the postpartum period is essential, not just for you but also for your baby. This section offers insights and holistic strategies to support your emotional health as you navigate this new chapter of life.

Many mothers experience change not only in their physical bodies but also in their emotional landscape and sense of identity. They may feel joy and gratitude, while also feeling exhausted. They're engaged and deeply bonded with their baby, yet overwhelmed and overstimulated. They may crave closeness while simultaneously longing for solitude.

This paradox of conflicting emotions is common, yet often misunderstood. Some may confuse it with "baby blues" or assume they're slipping into postpartum depression. But what many are actually experiencing is a natural period of transition—one that deserves to be acknowledged and supported.

Across cultures and generations, this transitional time has been honored in meaningful ways …

In Chinese culture, the tradition of Zuo Yuezi, or "sitting the month," offers rest and nourishment, helping the mother's energy to regain balance. In many Latin cultures, La Cuarentena refers to a forty-day period during which family members rally around the mother, providing both emotional and physical support. Similarly, in Indian tradition, postpartum mothers often return to the family home to be cared for and supported during this sacred time.

In contrast, Western culture tends to celebrate pregnancy and the birth itself yet often overlooks the importance of the postpartum experience.

In the 1970s, anthropologist Dana Raphael coined a term to capture this crucial phase of life: **Matrescence**. After studying over 250 cultures, she discovered that nearly all had rituals and practices meant to ease the mother's transition into parenthood.

Matrescence refers to the physical, psychological, and emotional changes a person undergoes while becoming a mother, from preconception through the postpartum period and beyond. And yes—*beyond*—because once you have a baby, you are forever postpartum. Your hormones will continue to shift, your emotions will ebb and flow, and your identity will evolve with each stage of your child's life.

There's power in naming things. I find strength in understanding the roots of words, their original meanings, their essence. Naming the unnamable gives you a sense of control over what once felt chaotic.

This confusing time of clashing emotions, unmet needs, and unrealistic expectations can make you feel like you're losing your mind. Those around you—family members, even other mothers—may not fully understand. If they never had a name for what they went through, they likely never developed a frame of reference to support you now.

In a time when everything can feel out of control, *having a name* for what you're going through can be grounding. It normalizes the postpartum experience and validates what you're feeling. It also opens the door for others to recognize that the postpartum period isn't just about bouncing back. It's a time of profound healing, growth, and transformation that deserves to be seen and honored.

A Celebration

Too often, it seems that postpartum is seen as opposite sides of a coin—a time of joyful bliss or a chore. It doesn't have to be. We can embrace the idea of "and" in the postpartum period. It is joyful *and* tiring. It is a new being *and* a loss of a way of life. It is inviting a new energy and life into your home *and* removing other energy and *possibly* people from your life. It is cause for celebration *and* sorrow. It is okay to experience *ands* in your postpartum journey. It is perfectly normal, perfectly human, perfectly matrescence.

SECTION I

Emotional Wellness and Mental Health

CHAPTER 1

UNDERSTANDING POSTPARTUM EMOTIONAL CHANGES

The postpartum period often brings a wide spectrum of emotions, ranging from overwhelming joy and love to uncertainty, anxiety, and deep fatigue. It's a transformative time. While many new mothers anticipate sleepless nights and physical recovery, the emotional shifts can catch them off guard.

One of the most common experiences in the days after childbirth is known as the **"baby blues."** According to the March of Dimes, about **4 in 5 women** experience the baby blues, typically beginning two to three days after giving birth and lasting up to two weeks. These emotional fluctuations are often due to a dramatic decrease in key reproductive and thyroid hormones, including estrogen and progesterone. As these hormones drop, it can lead to mood swings, tearfulness, irritability, and sadness.[1]

While the baby blues are common and temporary, it's important to pay close attention to how long symptoms last. If emotional difficulties persist or worsen after the two-week mark, it may be a sign of *postpartum depression* (PPD)—a more serious mental health condition that affects roughly 1 in 7 women, according to the American Psychological Association.[2] PPD requires compassionate support and often medical attention.

Your Mental Health Matters

After giving birth, mental health becomes essential, and yet, it can be one of the hardest areas to care for. You're adjusting to new routines, interrupted sleep, and the emotional toll of constant caregiving. Add to that the rollercoaster of hormonal changes, and it's easy to feel lost in your own body.

Many new mothers wonder, *"Are these emotions really mine, or are they just my hormones talking?"* The truth is that it's both. Hormonal fluctuations after birth play a significant role in shaping your emotional state, energy levels, and overall sense of well-being.

Understanding what's happening inside your body can be incredibly empowering. It helps normalize the experience and allows you to extend compassion to yourself during a time when you may be feeling most vulnerable.

The Postpartum Hormones You Should Know

Let's break down the key hormones involved in the postpartum transition and how they impact your physical and emotional health.

1. Prolactin: The Milk-Making Hormone

Prolactin levels rise significantly after birth to stimulate **milk production**. While it plays a crucial role in feeding your baby, it also impacts your mood. Increased prolactin is often accompanied by decreased estrogen and progesterone, which can contribute to low mood and fatigue.

Fun Fact: Prolactin also promotes nurturing behavior and helps reinforce the mother-baby bond.

2. Progesterone: The Calming Hormone

Progesterone drops sharply after delivery. This hormone, which supports pregnancy and has mood-stabilizing effects, can leave a noticeable gap in your emotional resilience once it declines.

Low progesterone is linked with:

- Depression or low mood
- Weight gain
- Gallbladder issues
- Sluggish thyroid function
- Decreased motivation for daily tasks like hygiene or cooking

This hormonal crash is one reason why previously enjoyable or manageable tasks can suddenly feel overwhelming.

3. Estrogen: The Multitasker

Like progesterone, estrogen also plunges after birth and remains low during breastfeeding. Estrogen plays a role in nearly every system of the body, including the brain.

Low estrogen may contribute to:

- Fatigue
- Vaginal dryness
- Joint pain
- Mood swings
- Low libido

- Hair loss
- Brain fog or difficulty concentrating

While these effects are temporary, they can feel frustrating and even isolating. Understanding their cause can reduce the guilt or confusion many mothers feel.

4. Oxytocin: The Love Hormone

Oxytocin spikes immediately after birth, especially during skin-to-skin contact and breastfeeding. It supports maternal bonding, emotional warmth, and can even ease physical pain.

It's sometimes called the "feel-good hormone" because of its role in elevating mood and reinforcing connection. Interestingly, its rise is directly tied to the drop in estrogen and progesterone. Nature's way of giving you a helping hand through the transition.

5. Testosterone: The Overlooked Ally

Though we don't often talk about it in the context of women, testosterone plays a big role in your postpartum experience. It helps regulate:

- Energy
- Mood
- Muscle mass
- Libido
- Fat metabolism

After childbirth, testosterone levels decline, which may add to feelings of exhaustion, decreased motivation, and body changes.

So, What Now? Finding Hope in the Chaos

If this all sounds overwhelming, take a deep breath. The good news is that understanding what's happening gives you power and perspective.

Your emotional ups and downs during the postpartum period are not signs of weakness. They are the body's response to an incredible physical and emotional shift. By recognizing these changes, you can offer yourself the grace, patience, and care you truly need.

You don't have to force yourself to feel "okay" all the time. Letting go of the need to be okay might just be the path to true healing.

The key is support—from yourself, your loved ones, your care providers, and your community. Whether it's talking to a friend, joining a postpartum group, or speaking with a therapist, every connection you make is a strand in the web that holds you up.

Coming Up Next

In the next chapter, we'll explore how to build a sustainable support network in the postpartum period—starting with family, friends, and care providers, and extending into community-based resources that can help you thrive, not just survive.

CHAPTER 2

BUILDING YOUR SUPPORT NETWORK

Why You Need a Support System During Postpartum Recovery

Having a support group during your postpartum recovery is essential for your mental and physical well-being. It's no exaggeration to say that no one should go through this time alone. As a new parent, no matter how many books you've read, videos you've watched, or doctor's appointments you've attended, you will still have questions, doubts, and moments of anxiety. You'll worry about your baby's well-being *and* your own. If you have older children, they're also entering a new phase. They're adjusting to a new sibling while continuing their own developmental journey.

All of this can be overwhelming. Without a support system to lean on, it can be exhausting at best, and at worst, detrimental to your health, your relationships, and your child(ren)'s development.

What *Is* a Support Network, Anyway?

Is it family? Friends? A group that meets once a week?
The answer: **Yes.** It can be any of those things—or all of them.

A network, by definition, is:

1. An arrangement of intersecting horizontal and vertical lines
2. A group or system of interconnected people or things

Your support network can be made up of people, places, or things—anything that intersects or connects with you and your needs. You are the nexus of these connections. Every business, school, organization, or group has a network. Think of them as built-in fail-safes.

One of my favorite shows is *Leverage*. In it, a character says, "My backup plans have backup plans." That line has always stuck with me.

I believe nothing on this planet functions without a network. Take the human brain, for example—it's made up of a vast network of synapses that connect information and stimuli to form pathways of learning, memory, and creativity. The more your neurons network, the more intelligent you become. The more your brain networks in a particular area, the stronger and more knowledgeable you become in that field. Eventually, with repetition and nurture, you become an expert—because that's what your brain has been trained to do.

So, how do you create these pathways? You nurture them.

Let's say you want to become an artist. You might start by reading books, watching videos, studying other artists, and eventually picking up a pencil or brush yourself. Over time, through practice and exposure, you develop your own expertise.

In the same way, building a support network—creating a supportive structure for a firm foundation in life—takes time, effort, and nurturing. Think of a spider's web. One strand might come undone easily in the wind, but a web with multiple strands intertwined is stronger than steel. It can withstand high winds. And we, too, must be able to withstand high winds—especially as we journey through the whirlwind of parenthood.

Our mental, physical, and spiritual well-being all depend on building these strong pathways.

So, how do you start nurturing a solid network?

Step one: Identify the kind of support you need.

Take stock of where you are right now. What drains you the most? What task exhausts you just thinking about it?

For me, it's cleaning. I used to love it. Honestly, I still do. But with kids, the house doesn't stay clean for long. I work long hours some weeks, and when I get home, all I want to do is get my steps in, help my son with his schoolwork, do my spiritual practice, and just relax. I mean, even writing that list feels like a workout! Adding cleaning to that lineup is overwhelming.

Ideally, I'd hire someone to come once a week to clean. Right now, I have someone come every three weeks to tackle the major areas of the house, and that makes a big difference.

Your situation may look different depending on where you are in your parenting journey. You may be pregnant and planning ahead, have older children, or already be in the thick of caring for a newborn. While planning ahead is always ideal, life rarely goes according to plan. Still, no matter where you are, you *can* nurture a network.

Let's begin with the first layer of that network: **the family**.

We'll imagine this network like a spider web—concentric circles and lines connecting the layers. At the center? You, the parent.

You can even sketch this out for yourself. We'll dive into how to do that later in the book.

Family as Support

Healthy family relationships are a strong source of connection. This is where traditions, stories, and history live. When you reach out to family, you gain insight, advice, and sometimes a space to vent. There are times when we just need a family member. I hear friends and clients frequently say, "I just needed to talk to my mom," and "I know what my dad would say, but I just needed to hear it," or "My Aunt Linda, she has the best way of saying things that just make me laugh."

I have found that even though I can go to friends, counselors, and peers for advice, there is something in the way my aunt says something that makes me feel good.

You might find out that your baby shares the same quirks or mannerisms you or a sibling had as a child. Maybe there are little tricks your mom, grandmother, or aunt used that *actually* work—and a few that didn't.

If healthy family ties aren't available to you, building a *chosen family* can be just as meaningful and beneficial.

Support Groups & Real-Life Friendships

When my firstborn was three, my husband was transferred to central Florida—not the theme park area, just regular ol' central Florida. I was completely alone. No friends, no family, nothing.

On top of that, we had moved from the concrete jungle of South Florida to a quiet, rural area. I felt like a fish out of water.

I didn't need help with the basics of childcare—I needed *people*. Friends I could talk to, vent to, and simply be around. I needed to feel less alone. So, I started looking for mom/toddler groups and found one that felt like a good fit.

We had weekly playdates at the park, activities at the local community center, and fun holiday events. I even met a mom who lived just a block away. Suddenly, I felt human again. I felt *sane*.

This is just one kind of support, but it made all the difference.

Types of Parenting and Community Groups

You can find local groups for just about every age and stage of your baby's life. There are:

- Mommy & Me classes
- Mother's Day Out programs
- Parenting circles and meetups
- Groups based on hobbies or lifestyle

In Nashville, there's a hiking group for parents of infants—they strap their babies into carriers and hit the trails at Warner Parks. These kinds of groups not only connect you to others, but they also help you get fresh air, exercise, and a dose of nature (which we know helps with stress and mood!)

You can also look into **non-parenting groups**. Maybe you love hiking, swimming, painting, or gardening. Hobbies can be an incredible way to stay connected to yourself—the person you were before parenthood, and the one you're still becoming.

These groups may not be your "in-the-trenches" crew, but they might just become the ones who bring you tea and muffins, hold the baby while you shower, or send that encouraging text when you need it most.

Why Peer Support Matters

We often underestimate how powerful it is to have someone who *gets it*.
Someone who's been there.
Someone who knows what it's like to be up all night, to question every decision, to feel the highs and lows of parenting.

Talking to other parents about the challenges you're facing—and hearing how they've handled similar situations—can offer perspective and relief. It also helps to have conversations around things like communication, routines, relationships, feeding, sleep, and even what's considered healthy vs. unhealthy behavior patterns.

And guess what? There are actual cognitive and emotional benefits to socializing:

- Reduced stress, depression, and anxiety
- Less loneliness
- Increased cognition and memory
- Improved long-term health and longevity

Support Outside of Parenting

The postpartum period can also bring up deeper emotional or relational challenges. It's a vulnerable time, and for some, it can be triggering.

For instance, it's not uncommon for partners to experience jealousy, resentment, or emotional withdrawal. Like moms, they may go through hormonal changes—but they may not realize what's causing their mood shifts. This can lead to depression, anger, or isolation.

Groups like Al-Anon or other 12-step and anonymous support programs offer confidential, safe spaces to talk. Members share phone numbers and offer support outside of meetings.

Local religious or spiritual organizations may also offer postpartum support, counseling, or social activities that can make you feel seen and connected.

Show Up for Your Support

The most important thing you can do? **Show up.** Whether it's a hobby group, a step program, a mommy-and-me circle, or a hiking meetup. Consistency is key. Investing time helps build trust and strengthens the relationships that will carry you through the hard days.

Practical Exercise: Mapping Your Support Network

Here is where you can sketch out your network or make a list if that makes more sense. Take a few moments to write down the people in your life you feel you can count on. Then divide them into categories:

- Can & want to call anytime
- Can call, but don't really want to unless necessary
- Can call in a crunch
- Emergency only

You can even go further and break it down by *task*:

- Help with cleaning, laundry, or food
- Ride to the doctor
- Trip to the grocery store
- Hold the baby while I shower/nap/breathe
- A shoulder to cry on

This can help you visualize the network we discussed earlier. I will briefly cover key highlights here. It will show you the support you already have and where there are gaps. You don't need a long list, but having just two or three people in your corner can ease so much of the pressure.

Final Thought

You are *not* weak or incapable for wanting a support network.
You were never meant to parent in isolation.
You should not be expected to carry it all alone.
That's not sustainable. And it's not safe—for you *or* your baby.

Now is the time to be honest about what you need. You deserve that!

Let's look at another aspect of postpartum emotional and mental health.

CHAPTER 3

RECOGNIZING YOUR EVOLVING IDENTITY

Losing and Rediscovering Myself After Motherhood

Can I recall my twenties? Some things I've forgotten, but others feel as fresh as yesterday. I remember being wide-eyed and new to the world. Working and making my own money, living in an apartment with roommates, finally able to make my own decisions. There were many long nights out with "friends" I barely knew, which often turned into early mornings. I remember sleeping. Yes—*I remember sleeping.*

Then I had my daughter. My firstborn. My life-changer. The late nights out were replaced by late nights awake with a colicky baby. Money was still being made, but it was spent on pacifiers, diapers, baby clothes, and toys. Decisions were still being made, but suddenly, every choice impacted this brand-new little person in my life.

A few years later, my son came along. And just like that, I had two little ones constantly at the forefront of my thoughts.

I experienced postpartum hyperthyroidism after both of my pregnancies. The first time, it was a complete shock. I had no idea what was happening to me until my mother-in-law recognized the signs. She had gone through it herself and helped me understand that I was dealing with another hormone change.

Physically, my body went through dramatic changes. I gained a lot of weight, then lost it. Mentally, I went from feeling depressed during pregnancy to loving motherhood—while also being completely exhausted. As a preschool teacher, I thought I knew nearly everything about babies and young children. But when it came to raising my own child, I quickly realized I was starting from scratch.

I was blindsided by the overwhelming uncertainty. Was I doing anything right? And then came the fear—deep, paralyzing fear that something might happen to my baby. That he might get hurt, or worse.

I thought I was prepared. But nothing could have prepared me for the unpreparable—my mental state, my emotional shifts, and the sensation that the solid ground I once stood on had vanished.

Identity Crisis After Birth

So much of my identity had been tied to my profession as a teacher. When I realized I couldn't easily apply those skills to parenting, I felt like a failure. I no longer knew who I was in this new relationship—with my child or with myself. I had also been a writer, but once the baby came, I could barely find time to write. My only remaining hobby was reading, and even that became a rare occurrence.

In what felt like the blink of an eye, everything I had been—professionally, mentally, creatively—was gone. My confidence disappeared. My sense of accomplishment, of capability, of self ... all vanished.

It *did* get better, eventually. But it took a long time.

Now I know this is common. It happens to many new parents—not just the birthing parent, but also partners, siblings, friends, and relatives. Sometimes, you don't notice it until well after the medical postpartum period. Maybe even years later. The ground shifts. Your identity feels shaken.

What Are Some Signs This Might Be Happening to You?

Do you find yourself mourning the life you had before pregnancy?
Do you struggle to describe who you are now that you're a mother?
Do you feel like you're taking care of everyone else except yourself?

How do you navigate the loss of self—or the transformation of who you once were?

1. Acceptance

Start with acceptance. Accept that you've gone through a profound change—physically, emotionally, mentally, and even spatially. Your relationship with your environment is different now.

Where you once walked into the kitchen at midnight for a glass of water, now you're tiptoeing in to store your pumped breast milk. Where you once stayed up late for fun, now it's because your baby needs you. Life has changed. You may feel unsteady. That's normal.

2. Old and New Hobbies

Just because you've changed doesn't mean you've lost value. In fact, you have an opportunity to reinvent yourself.

You don't have to enjoy the same things you did before. Maybe something you never liked now brings comfort and connection. Yes—try to make space for your old hobbies. But also be open to discovering new ones.

For me, writing and reading were my go-to hobbies. However, when my daughter showed an interest in art, I started painting. I never considered myself artistic. Now I love it. I enjoy making installation art and coloring, just for the joy of it.

My son introduced me to puzzle games. Together we play cards, chess, and checkers. I rediscovered word searches and crossword puzzles. Later, I discovered walking, and then hiking. It became a hobby I could maintain even with children in tow. My writing shifted too—less fiction, more journaling and nonfiction.

Think about what you might try: painting, hiking, ice skating, running, bowling, joining a book club. You might just surprise yourself.

3. Wait on the Weight

Our bodies are another core part of identity. And after pregnancy, the relationship we have with our bodies often changes.

Some people develop body dysmorphia—a serious condition that causes distorted self-perception. But even without that diagnosis, it's common to wish you could just "bounce back" to your pre-pregnancy self.

Instead of focusing on the past, try to marvel at what your body has accomplished. You created life. You may be lactating. Your body expanded and contracted, and now continues to carry you through each day. Celebrate what you *can* do—get out of bed, take a walk, pick up your baby. These small wins are huge.

Reframing your thoughts this way builds self-esteem and nurtures a more loving self-identity.

4. Real Self-Care

I often mention self-care in my writing—not because it's trendy, but because it's essential. And I don't mean massages or manicures (although those are great too). I mean the basics:

- Brush your teeth
- Shower
- Comb your hair
- Moisturize your skin

As you care for your body, talk kindly to it. I silently thank each part: *I love my legs. I'm proud of what you do. Thank you, arms.* I don't say it aloud—my kids would probably think I'm being a little "woo-woo," but the practice grounds me. It's about creating a gentle, positive narrative for yourself.

5. Stop Comparing

Everyone has their idea of what it means to be a "good parent" or a "good woman." Your identity isn't defined by society's checklists.

What makes *you* feel like a good mother? What makes you feel loved, cared for, and beautiful? These answers are yours alone.

You're part of a long lineage of parents, yet your approach is unique and valid.

You don't have to follow every trend. You don't need diamond earrings or a spa day to prove your worth.

A therapist once said, "Be a good enough parent most of the time." I love that. You can apply it to everything: be a good enough partner, writer, daughter, friend—most of the time. That's enough. No one gets it right 100% of the time.

Give Yourself Grace

Motherhood transforms your sense of self. It's natural to feel lost for a while. But you *will* find your footing again. Be patient with yourself as your identity evolves.

Keep engaging in things that make you feel whole, whether old hobbies or new discoveries. Speak to yourself with love. Try one new thing at a time. Give yourself grace. You are not less—you are becoming.

Experiencing a shift in identity after childbirth is a common and natural part of becoming a parent. This transition—*matrescence*—involves significant emotional, physical, and social changes. While some degree of identity adjustment is expected, it's important to recognize when these feelings become overwhelming and may require professional support.

When to Seek Help

Consider reaching out to a mental health professional if you experience:

- Persistent feelings of sadness, anxiety, or hopelessness that last more than two weeks

- Difficulty bonding with your baby or feeling detached from your child
- Loss of interest in activities you once enjoyed
- Changes in appetite or sleep patterns unrelated to your baby's schedule
- Thoughts of self-harm or harming your baby

These symptoms may indicate postpartum depression (PPD), which affects approximately 10 to 20 percent of new mothers. PPD can occur anytime within the first year after childbirth and is distinct from the "baby blues," which typically resolve within two weeks.

Additionally, suppose you're struggling with a sense of lost identity, feeling overwhelmed by the demands of motherhood, or experiencing significant stress in your relationships or daily functioning. In that case, it's advisable to seek support.

Where to Find Support

- **Postpartum Support International (PSI):** Offers resources and a helpline (1-800-944-4773) for new parents experiencing mental health challenges.
- **National Alliance on Mental Illness (NAMI):** Provides information and support groups for individuals dealing with mental health conditions, including postpartum issues (1-800-950-6264).
- **Substance Abuse and Mental Health Services Administration (SAMHSA):** Offers a 24/7 helpline (1-800-662-HELP) and resources for finding mental health services.

Remember, seeking help is a sign of strength, not weakness. Early intervention can lead to better outcomes for both you and your baby. If you're in Nashville, Tennessee, and need assistance finding local resources, feel free to ask me. Email me at ghenetleeyong@gmail.com

CHAPTER 4

MINDFULNESS AND MENTAL HYGIENE FOR NEW PARENTS

Incorporating mindfulness techniques into your daily routine can significantly enhance emotional well-being, especially during the early postpartum period. Practices such as meditation, deep breathing, and gentle yoga help ground you in the present moment, reduce anxiety, and promote relaxation. These activities not only support your mental health but also foster a deeper connection with yourself and your baby, creating a calm and nurturing environment at home.

Why Mindfulness Matters After Birth

The postpartum period is a time of profound transition. Beyond the rapid hormonal and chemical shifts in your body, you're adjusting to new schedules, endless to-do lists, feeding routines, diaper changes, and doctors' appointments. Some days are filled with visitors, and others may feel lonely and isolated. It can be overwhelming. Staying balanced may seem impossible, but it's not.

Things may not always go according to plan. Birth experiences vary widely, and the emotional impact of how your baby enters the world can be significant. I remember the day I had a C-section—how proud I felt, yet how quickly that pride was dampened by the words of others. One person said, "Oh, but you didn't *really* give birth. You had a C-section." Their words stung, and for a moment, I questioned my experience. But let me say this clearly: *every birth is a birth.*

A Cesarean section (C-section) is a common (and sometimes life-saving) surgical procedure in which a baby is delivered through incisions in the abdomen and uterus. It may be planned for medical reasons—like placenta previa, breech presentation, or a previous C-section—or arise unexpectedly during labor due to complications such as fetal distress or stalled progression. Physically, recovery from a C-section can take longer than a vaginal birth, involving wound care, limited mobility, and several weeks of healing.

But the emotional and mental health aspects of a C-section are just as vital to acknowledge. For some parents, especially those who had envisioned a vaginal birth, an unplanned C-section can bring feelings of grief, disappointment, guilt, or even failure. These emotions can fuel anxiety, depression, or a sense of disconnection—particularly if immediate bonding is delayed or breastfeeding becomes more difficult. Social stigma or unsolicited comments can intensify these feelings, leaving new parents confused or ashamed. This is why emotional validation, gentle support, and open conversations are essential. Talking with a therapist, postpartum doula, or support group can help you process your experience and feel seen as the courageous, resilient parent you are.

Practicing proper mental hygiene, such as simple, intentional actions that support emotional well-being, can help you maintain equilibrium and boost your resilience. Whether you're taking five quiet minutes to breathe, journaling your thoughts, or asking for help when you need it, these small efforts build a foundation of strength, self-awareness, and healing.

Mental Hygiene Practices for the Postpartum Journey

1. Talk, Talk, Talk

Sharing your feelings out loud is one of the most healing things you can do. Whether it's a friend, therapist, partner, spiritual advisor, or fellow parent, having someone to listen to you is essential.

According to the American Psychological Association[2], social connection is a protective factor for mental health. Speaking openly can help organize your thoughts, reduce stress, and provide validation. Something every new parent deserves.

You might also consider joining a postpartum support group. These spaces can be invaluable, offering understanding, shared experiences, and emotional relief.

2. Take Micro Breaks

Even just 2 to 3 minutes away from the constant demands of caregiving can make a difference. When the baby is safe and settled, set a timer and allow yourself to:

- Breathe deeply using the Box Breathing method (4 seconds in, 4 seconds hold, 4 seconds out, 4 seconds hold again)
- Do a few jumping jacks or a quick stretch
- Try a simple lymphatic massage for circulation and tension relief. This is a specific type of massage geared toward helping move fluid through your lymphatic system, helping to flush out toxins. It is a light-touch massage

and can be self-applied. (I will put a link in Appendix II - Resources.)

These quick resets calm the nervous system, increase focus, and support emotional regulation.

3. Take a Walk

Getting outside is one of the best things you can do for your mind and body. A 2020 review published in *Frontiers in Psychology* confirms that walking in nature reduces stress, boosts mood, and enhances well-being.[3]

Walk alone or with your baby in a carrier or stroller. The fresh air, gentle movement, and shift in scenery can soothe both you and your child. Morning light helps regulate your circadian rhythm and may improve sleep quality. This is something every new parent needs!

4. Eat (Yes, Eat!) and Nourish Your Brain

Postpartum moms often forget to eat—especially in the chaos of mornings and cluster feedings. Prioritize **nutrient-dense, easy-access meals and snacks** throughout the day.

Try:

- Ready-to-go veggie trays and fruit (berries, bananas, grapes)
- Lean proteins: eggs, turkey, chicken, tofu, lentils
- Whole grains and healthy fats: avocado toast, hummus with crackers
- Hydration: water, herbal teas, and smoothies

According to Harvard Health, good nutrition is vital for postpartum recovery and mental health. It impacts energy, hormone regulation, and even mood.[4]

5. Play Soft, Calming Music

Gentle instrumental or nature-inspired music can ease tension, help you focus, and calm your baby. Research from Stanford University shows that music can lower blood pressure, slow heart rate, and reduce cortisol levels (the stress hormone).[5]

Choose playlists with soothing melodies and keep the volume low. Over time, this can become a cue for calm and regulation—for both you and your baby.

6. Practice Deep Breathing

A simple breathing technique can work wonders. Here's a story:

> One day, when I was overwhelmed and venting to my mentor, she gently said, "Take a deep breath in. And out." I wanted to roll my eyes (I might have ... we were on the phone), but I trusted her. She had me do it several times. Then she asked, "Are your hands clenched?" They were. "Open them. Feel the air." I did. I kept walking, breathing, and slowly began to relax. Within minutes, I felt lighter.

Breathing sends signals to the parasympathetic nervous system—the part of your body that says, "You're safe." It boosts oxygen to your brain, improves circulation, and helps with clear thinking. Even just one minute of focused breathing can help you reset.

7. Try Affirmations

Affirmations are simple, empowering statements that can help shift your mindset. According to *Psychology Today*, repeated positive affirmations may reduce stress, improve confidence, and reinforce desired behaviors through a phenomenon called **self-affirmation theory***.[6]

Tailor your affirmations to be personal and realistic. Here are a few to try:

- "I am learning to care for myself as I care for others."
- "I take small steps toward balance every day."
- "I'm proud of what I accomplished today."
- "I allow myself grace during this time of change."

8. Build a Meditative Moment

Meditation doesn't have to be long or complicated. In the early postpartum weeks, it may be a moment of silence, a breath practice, a few affirmations, or simply closing your eyes and listening to soft music.

Even three to five minutes of mindfulness can reduce stress and improve your mood. Apps like Insight Timer, Calm, or Expectful offer free meditations tailored to new parents.

9. Accept Help (Seriously, Say Yes)

If someone offers to help, let them. Whether it's holding the baby, doing the dishes, or grabbing groceries, say yes.

Accepting help is not a weakness. It's wise. A 2021 study in *BMC Pregnancy and Childbirth* showed that postpartum moms with more perceived support had lower levels of depression and anxiety.[7] Help builds your village and gives you a chance to rest, recover, and recharge.

10. Treat Yourself Like You Matter (Because You Do)

Did you survive a night of cluster feeding (baby feeding in short, consecutive sessions)? Get the toddler out the door? Make yourself a sandwich?

Celebrate it.

You deserve moments of joy and self-appreciation. Whether it's five minutes with a favorite show, a special snack, skincare, or a walk with your favorite drink, do something that tells your brain, "You're doing great."

Validation is not vanity. It's survival.

Another helpful activity to try is journaling. There are evidence-based benefits to journaling, and it's commonly used as a therapeutic practice. The next chapter will explore this practice in depth.

*Links located in Appendix: Resources.

CHAPTER 5

JOURNALING FOR EMOTIONAL CLARITY

Writing down your thoughts and feelings can be a therapeutic way to process the myriad of emotions that accompany new motherhood. Journaling allows you to express fears, joys, and uncertainties, providing clarity and a sense of release. It also serves as a personal record of your journey, highlighting growth and resilience.

Journaling is extensively researched. Studies show that journaling has actual, measurable benefits. According to NIH*, a study conducted on seventy people with varying medical conditions, journaling "was associated with decreased mental distress and increased well-being relative to baseline." It was also "associated with less depressive symptoms and anxiety after 1 month and greater resilience after the first and second month, relative to usual care."[8]

Journaling can help in ways that meditation alone cannot. Getting your thoughts down on paper gives you a way to visually see the pattern of your thoughts and clearly identify areas of improvement or of amplification. Let's look at ways journaling has been proven to help with mental health. Then we will look at different types of journaling and how to implement those in your life. You can also narrow down on what could work for you at different stages in your life.

Benefits of Journaling

Organize Thoughts

Journaling is a powerful tool for organizing thoughts because it allows you to slow down and give structure to the ideas and emotions swirling in your mind. By putting pen to paper, you create a space to process experiences, clarify feelings, and break down complex problems into manageable parts. This practice helps identify patterns, set intentions, and prioritize what truly matters. Over time, journaling can bring a sense of order and calm, making it easier to make decisions and respond to challenges with clarity and confidence.

Pros and Cons

Journaling is a helpful way to explore the pros and cons of any decision or situation because it encourages honest and thoughtful reflection. When you write things down, you can separate emotions from facts and lay out the benefits and drawbacks more clearly. This process helps you see the full picture—what you might gain, what you could lose, and how each outcome aligns with your values or goals. Journaling also gives you space to consider long-term effects and imagine how different choices might make you feel over time. By organizing your thoughts on paper, you're more likely to make balanced, informed decisions with greater confidence.

Positive Self-Validation

Journaling can be a powerful tool for positive self-validation by giving you a space to acknowledge your strengths, achievements, and personal growth. Writing about your experiences allows you to recognize the effort you've put in, celebrate small wins, and affirm your worth without needing external approval. With consistent repetition, this practice helps build a stronger, more compassionate inner voice that reminds you of your value, even during challenging moments. By regularly reflecting on what you're proud of or how you've overcome obstacles, journaling reinforces self-belief and creates a habit of uplifting and encouraging yourself from within.

Track Emotions

Journaling is an effective way to track emotions because it provides a consistent space to express and reflect on how you feel and how those feelings may or may not change. By writing regularly, you can begin to notice patterns in your mood, triggers for certain emotions, and how different situations affect your mental well-being. This awareness can lead to deeper self-understanding and make it easier to manage stress, improve relationships, or seek support when needed. Over time, reviewing past journal entries can reveal growth, resilience, and shifts in perspective, helping you better navigate future emotional experiences with clarity and confidence.

Track Your Milestones and Look Back at How Far You've Come

Journaling is a meaningful way to track your personal milestones and reflect on how far you've come. By recording your thoughts, goals, and experiences over time, you create a written timeline of your journey, capturing both the challenges you've faced and the progress you've made. Looking back on past entries allows you to see growth that might otherwise go unnoticed, reminding you of the strength, resilience, and lessons gained along the way. This perspective can be deeply encouraging, especially during difficult chapters in life, as it reinforces your ability to overcome obstacles and continue moving forward with purpose and confidence.

Types of Journaling

Realistically, not everyone can journal for hours at a time. And, to be completely honest, ten minutes might be pushing it. Utilizing different types of journaling can help you incorporate journaling into your life in a way that fits your needs so you can get the benefits it provides. We will go through different types of journaling to see how you can fit this into your schedule.

Traditional

Traditional journaling involves writing by hand in a notebook or diary, offering a personal and tactile experience that encourages deep reflection and connection with your thoughts. This form of journaling often feels more intimate and intentional, allowing you to slow down and be fully present as you express your emotions, record daily events, or explore inner thoughts. The physical act of writing can enhance memory and emotional processing, making it easier to sort through feelings or gain clarity on complex situations. For many, traditional journaling becomes a cherished routine—a quiet moment of self-care that nurtures mindfulness, creativity, and personal growth. This type of journaling can take several minutes to hours to do. While extremely therapeutic, this is time-intensive and may not be practical all the time.

Bullet

Bullet journaling is a customizable and efficient method of organizing your thoughts, tasks, and goals using a simple system of symbols, lists, and short-form entries. Unlike traditional journaling, which often involves long, reflective writing, bullet journaling uses bullet points to capture information quickly and clearly. This method can include daily to-do lists, habit trackers, mood logs, goal-setting pages, and creative elements like doodles or quotes. Its flexibility allows you to design a system that fits your lifestyle, making it both a planner and a personal journal. Bullet journaling helps improve focus, time management, and mindfulness by keeping everything in one thoughtfully organized place.

Poem

Writing poetry can be a beautiful way to express how you feel during the postpartum period. It offers a creative outlet to capture the beauty, vulnerability, and complexity of this transformative time. Like journaling, poetry becomes a gentle companion, holding space for your joys, fears, and shifting identity. Through a few honest lines or a flowing verse, you can give voice to emotions that may feel too heavy or tangled to speak aloud. In this way, poetry becomes both reflection and release, helping you process your experience and connect more deeply with yourself.

There is no good or bad poetry when journaling this way. There is just you, your thoughts, and your emotions on the page. No need for explanations or solutions. Just the raw, visual version of your inner world unfolding in words.

Here is something I wrote when my son was four months old:

Tired

Day and night. I am tired in my sleep.

I dream tired dreams.

> When I wake, I walk—one foot in front of the other—longing, waiting for ...
>
> The baby is crying. The baby is hungry.
>
> K needs help with homework.
>
> I am in it deep.
>
> When will I ever sleep?
>
> I walk one foot in front of the other—longing, waiting for ...

Life during that time was financially difficult. With only my husband working, a five year old in school, and just one car, our resources were stretched thin. I couldn't afford aftercare, and I was exhausted. So, I wrote because I couldn't always express what I was feeling in clear, concise language. But putting words on paper helped me process emotions I couldn't yet name.

Drawing

Drawing is another powerful form of journaling, especially during the postpartum period when words may feel out of reach. Through simple sketches, colors, or shapes, you can express emotions, tell stories, and mark moments that might be difficult to put into language. Drawing allows you to slow down and connect with your inner world visually and intuitively. It doesn't have to be artistic or polished—what matters is the feeling behind each line or image. Whether you're doodling during nap time or creating symbolic illustrations of your experience, drawing offers a quiet space to process, reflect, and heal.

Micro-Journaling

The power of micro-journaling lies in its brevity and simplicity. It can help you stay focused, grounded, and productive without overwhelming your day. This form of journaling is ideal for those who find clarity and calm in setting daily intentions. Simply choose three areas you want to focus on, write them down, and you're done. For example, your focus points might be:

1. Speak words of kindness to myself
2. Allow myself time
3. Spend five minutes in solitude

These goals are intentionally self-focused, helping you nurture your well-being so you can show up as your best self for your family. Micro-journaling encourages mindfulness, supports emotional balance, and offers a simple structure to guide your day. It is perfect whether you're new to journaling or just looking for a quick, effective practice.

Note-taking/Post-it

I love this method of journaling because it's so simple and spontaneous. You just leave yourself little notes throughout the day—on whatever you have handy: notebooks, planners, grocery lists, or scraps of paper. You might jot down phrases like *I've got this, Take a breath, I made an awesome lunch,* or *I handled that tantrum like a pro.* Even tender observations like *I love the smell of the baby's clothes* or *I love the way she holds my hand while nursing* can become meaningful reminders of your daily joys.

Capturing these small moments and offering yourself encouragement is a gentle yet powerful way to lift your mood, build confidence, and invite more smiles into your day. I even like to write little affirmations in my planner—I forget about them until I stumble across them later in the year, and it always feels like a kind word from my past self.

Speech to Text/Voice Recording

Speech-to-text or voice-recording journaling is a wonderful option for those moments when your hands are full or your thoughts are flowing too quickly to write them down. Especially during the postpartum period, when time and energy are limited, speaking your thoughts aloud can feel more natural and accessible. You can record voice notes on your phone or use speech-to-text apps to capture your reflections, emotions, or daily experiences.

This method allows you to process feelings in real time, whether you're nursing, walking, or simply lying down with your baby. It's less about polished words and more about honest expression—freeing your mind without the pressure of grammar or structure. Later, you can choose to transcribe or reflect on these recordings, or simply let them stand as audio snapshots of your journey.

Night or Day

Journaling can be powerful in the morning or at night—it all depends on what feels right for you. Morning journaling helps set the tone for your day, offering clarity, intention, and a sense of purpose before the busyness begins. It's a chance to reflect on how you want to show up and what you want to focus on. On the other hand, nighttime journaling offers space to wind down, release lingering thoughts, and process the day's events. It can promote better sleep by clearing mental clutter and helping you acknowledge small wins or emotions that come up.

There's no "right" time—just the time that best fits your rhythm. Some people thrive on morning reflection, while others find comfort in ending the day with pen in hand. The key is consistency and choosing a time that supports your well-being.

No matter how you choose to journal—whether it's through poetry, lists, voice notes, or simple scribbles—doing so can greatly improve your mental health, help you gain clarity, and reduce anxiety. Journaling is a deeply personal practice. What matters most is creating space to check in with yourself, honor your experiences, and express your truth without judgment. As a new parent, your days may feel full and unpredictable, but even a few moments of reflection can offer grounding and peace. Be gentle with yourself, stay curious, and let your journaling practice evolve with you.

Sometimes, no matter how well you integrate mindfulness into your routines or how hard you try on your own, there are emotional states that you may not be able to overcome without support. The following chapter will explore these challenges and discuss when it's time to seek help.

CHAPTER 6

SEEKING PROFESSIONAL SUPPORT WHEN NEEDED

If feelings of sadness, anxiety, or overwhelm become persistent or interfere with daily functioning, seeking professional support is crucial. Mental health professionals specializing in postpartum care can provide tailored strategies and interventions to support your emotional health. Remember, reaching out is a sign of strength and an important step in caring for both yourself and your baby.

When is it time to reach out for professional help? The simple answer is whenever you want to. You do not have to be experiencing a crisis to reach out for help. Getting help is better the earlier you get it. Let's look at some indicators that may help you make a decision.

Many new moms experience a period of emotional ups and downs. As previously mentioned, this is often called the "baby blues" and is very common (up to 80 percent of new moms).

Normal Postpartum "Baby Blues":

- Usually starts within the first *two to three days* after birth
- Peaks around day *four or five*
- Resolves on its own by *two weeks* postpartum

Common feelings include:

- Tearfulness for no clear reason
- Mood swings
- Feeling overwhelmed
- Irritability
- Trouble sleeping (even when baby is sleeping)
- Mild anxiety

These symptoms can feel intense but are usually short-lived and manageable with support, rest, and reassurance.

What's Not Normal: Signs of Postpartum Depression (PPD)

PPD affects **one in seven moms** (and can even affect partners too).

When to be concerned:

- Symptoms last longer than two weeks
- Symptoms interfere with daily functioning or bonding with baby
- The intensity of emotions feels overwhelming or unshakable

PPD Symptoms Can Include:

- Persistent sadness or hopelessness
- Loss of interest in things you used to enjoy

- Extreme fatigue or lack of energy
- Feelings of worthlessness, shame, or guilt
- Difficulty bonding with your baby
- Withdrawing from loved ones
- Anxiety or panic attacks
- Changes in appetite or sleep (not just from baby)
- Thoughts of harming yourself or your baby (this needs immediate help)

Also Important: Other Postpartum Mood Disorders

- **Postpartum Anxiety:** excessive worry, restlessness, racing thoughts
- **Postpartum OCD:** intrusive, unwanted thoughts or mental images often related to baby safety
- **Postpartum Psychosis** (very rare): hallucinations, delusions, confusion (a medical emergency)

What to Do if You're not Sure

- **Talk to someone:** your provider, a doula, or a therapist
- **You are not alone:** Support is out there
- **Treatment works:** therapy, support groups, sometimes medication

By acknowledging and addressing your emotional needs during the postpartum period, you lay the foundation for a balanced and fulfilling motherhood journey. Embrace the support available to you, and remember that caring for yourself is integral to caring for your child.

Soon, the baby will sleep longer and become more independent. You will once again be able to tell dawn from dusk, and your energy will come back. As the saying goes, "this too shall pass." Try to enjoy the small moments and know things will get better. If you begin experiencing longer and darker moods, please speak to your physician who can help point you in the right direction for professional help. There is NO shame in getting help, only relief.

NATURE IMMERSION

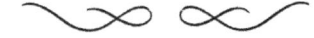

STEP ONE - OBSERVE

Definition: 1) Notice or perceive something and register it as being significant 2) Make a remark

This week, take time to observe—not just the world around you but yourself.

During pregnancy, you likely spent a lot of time noticing changes in your body. You observed your home, considering how its design and items would affect your little one. You watched older children, imagining how they would interact with the baby. You may have studied your spouse and family, wondering how their roles and relationships would shift. And, of course, you observed the world at large—how safe, supportive, or challenging it might be for your growing family.

But in all of this, did you take time to observe yourself? Not as a parent, not in relation to others, but simply as *you*?

Now, with your baby earthside, you may still be carrying the weight of those observations, noticing the scars, the loose skin, the exhaustion, the expectations. The feeling of being everything for someone else.

This week is about observation—of nature and yourself. How do you interact with nature? How do you feel about it? And how do you interact with yourself? How do you feel about *you*?

These aren't easy questions, and there are no right or wrong answers. Be honest. Your responses are simply a reflection of this moment in time. The more you practice observing the natural world without judgment, the more you can learn to observe yourself with greater compassion.

Walking Nature Reflection and Activity

Go for a walk (you can take the baby/children with you). If at all possible, try to go alone. Spend five to ten minutes walking at an easy pace. Observe nature around you—trees, bushes, hedges, rocks, sky, wind, squirrels, chipmunks, etc. Notice the colors, textures, sounds, and movements. Observe your initial reactions to these components in nature.

Alternative

Not all of us can simply step outside for a walk whenever we want. If you've had a complicated birth or pregnancy, even the thought of going out can feel overwhelming. You may also live in an area where walking doesn't feel safe or comfortable. I remember when I first started walking for weight loss, I wasn't comfortable walking in my neighborhood. While I had the option of going to a park, it wasn't always possible.

If getting outside isn't an option, you can still connect with nature from your porch, backyard, or balcony. Take a few moments to sit and do a nature reflection, noticing the sky, the trees, or even a potted plant nearby. If you'd like to incorporate movement, try walking in place.

LIIT (Low Impact Interval Training): Windmills

Part of recovering involves movement. While walking is a great cardio and overall exercise, and it helps to connect you with nature if done outdoors, sometimes more targeted work is needed to contract and strengthen muscles that were stretched out over the last nine months. Depending on your birthing experience, you may not be able to do more than walk for several weeks after giving birth.

Introducing LIIT (low impact interval training) is a great way to ease back into larger muscle work and strengthening. These exercises can be done outdoors in your backyard or at the park, in a field, or on the beach, wherever your nature is. Doing them outdoors adds to their effectiveness as you gain the benefits from grounding, getting vitamin D from the sun (safely), and breathing in fresh air and the organic compounds carried by the wind.

This low-impact exercise engages your core, helps to increase balance by crossing the meridian line, provides a great stretch, and can be easily adjusted based on your energy level. It also begins in a power pose, perfect for when you need a boost of confidence and strength!

Stand with your arms stretched out to the sides. Bend at the waist, reaching your fingertips toward the opposite toes. Remember to only bend or reach as far as it's comfortable. DO NOT strain yourself. Return to standing and repeat on the other side. Continue alternating for a total of five repetitions on each side. Complete two sets.

To modify the exercise, you can slow down your pace or perform the movement in a seated position, keeping an upright posture. If you want to increase the intensity, move faster or add more sets.

To modify the exercise further, lie flat on your back, keep bent in a dead bug position, and do the windmill motion, reaching across your body to touch your opposite knee or foot. You do not need to lift your head or perform a crunch, as this can add unnecessary pressure to the pelvic floor. Even small movements can help restore energy and connection.

Whether modified or not, pay attention to your body. Breathe in to raise up and out to bend. Engage your core by pulling your belly button in. Do the motions slowly and controlled. If you experience pain or discomfort, STOP. There is no race. Recovery takes time, and so does strengthening your muscles.

Mindfulness Breath Practice

Pay attention to your breath. Take full breaths and exhale completely. For example, if you breathe in for five seconds, then breathe out for five seconds. Try to do this for a minute, even as your pace increases. I learned this technique from a retired Green Beret. It's how they can do long marches with heavy sacks for so long before needing to rest. The idea is that you are getting a steady intake of oxygen and training your body to regulate your breathing as your heart rate increases. In turn, endurance increases, allowing you to spend longer periods of time in exercises such as walking, working out, cleaning, etc.

Dietary Focus - Soups

During postpartum recovery, digestion can be sensitive, and gas can easily accumulate in the gut. If you've had a C-section, being mindful of what you eat is even more important, as the incision site can make bloating and stomach discomfort more painful. Heavy or greasy foods may cause digestive upset, making it essential to choose nourishing meals that are easy on the stomach.

Soups are an excellent option during this time. They provide hydration, essential nutrients, and warmth, all while being gentle on your digestion. They're also easy to prepare in advance, making them perfect for meal prep—you can freeze individual portions and reheat them for a quick, nourishing meal.

One of my favorite postpartum soups is homemade ramen. Unlike store-bought ramen, which is often loaded with sodium and preservatives, making it from scratch allows you to use high-quality noodles and add healing ingredients like bone broth, fresh vegetables, garlic, and ginger—foods that support recovery, boost immunity, and promote overall well-being

*See appendix for recipes

Journal Questions

Documenting your feelings and emotions around food can help you identify underlying scripts you have *been told* and *told yourself* over the years. It can also help you associate positive emotions and memories with certain foods. I loved it when I would see my mother take out the flour and the large soup pot. That always meant that she was going to put these large dumplings in the soup, a favorite of mine and my siblings. We sat in the kitchen and talked while she prepped, and we asked a thousand times when it would be ready. No matter what type of day we had, the smells and anticipation of those big drop dumplings lifted our spirits. Do you have a favorite memory surrounding soup? If not, can you introduce a new tradition to your family?

Step One - Observe

How do you currently connect with nature in your daily life? Do you have houseplants, a garden, or pets? Do you spend time outdoors, even in small ways?

Step One - Observe

Reflect on what you observed during your walk or time outdoors. How did it make you feel? There's no right or wrong answer here—just acknowledgment. If the sound of birds was soothing, note that. If a squirrel startled you or made you uncomfortable, write it down. This exercise is about honest reflection, free of judgment, simply recognize your feelings as they are.

Step One - Observe

Artist Within ~ Observe Without Expectation

Create artwork that captures the experience of being seen without expectation. Just as nature exists without seeking approval—trees grow, rivers flow, the sky shifts—how can you depict yourself in a way that embraces change without judgment? Consider using organic forms, layers, or natural textures to express the contrast between self-perception and the effortless presence of nature. Creating art should be enjoyable. As you work, release expectations on how your piece "should" look or what someone else may think of it. You have the right to freely create without judgment.

SECTION II

Physical Recovery and Self-Care

CHAPTER 7

THE FOURTH TRIMESTER: A LOOK AT TRADITIONAL AND CULTURAL PRACTICES AROUND HYGIENE

The initial weeks following childbirth, often referred to as the "fourth trimester," involve significant physical adjustments as your body recovers. Common experiences include uterine contractions as it returns to its pre-pregnancy size, perineal discomfort, and hormonal fluctuations. Recognizing these changes as natural parts of the healing process can help you navigate this period with greater ease.

Nurturing your body during the postpartum period is crucial for a smooth recovery and overall well-being. This section offers holistic strategies to support your physical healing and self-care journey after childbirth.

It's interesting to look at traditional practices in postpartum care and compare them to what we know today. How has traditional practice stood up to modern medicine and knowledge? Are there traditional practices that can still be followed? What is the reasoning for certain postpartum traditions? In this chapter, we will look at some of those traditions and list some important hygiene postpartum care practices for you to follow.

Some of the traditional themes across various cultures is the eating of warm foods in the first month of recovery, staying home, limiting activity (including cleaning), not bathing, using only boiled water, not brushing teeth, and limiting visitors to the home.

Eating Warm Foods

Then: The reasoning behind this tradition is that it is thought that healing happens through warmth, and cold food could introduce stomach upset and cause healing to take longer. There was also the belief that cold foods such as fruits and vegetables could cause diarrhea and gas. Traditionally, warm foods consisted of high-protein options such as chicken, duck, fish, and tofu, depending on the area.

Now: The modern recommendation is to avoid cold foods after birth for four to six weeks because the body needs nutrient-dense foods that are easy to digest. Cold foods could temporarily slow down digestive enzymes and may also cause severely painful gas which could be especially unpleasant after having a C-section. That is why cooked foods high in nutrients are the best to ingest in the first month after birth. Avoiding foods that are harsh on the digestive system will decrease painful gas and bloating and increase the rate of recovery.

Stay Home

Then: Traditionally, it was encouraged to stay home for up to thirty days after the baby was born. In fact, some cultures went as far as to say that mom should stay in her room for those thirty days and in bed for the first two weeks. The idea is that the new mother and baby are susceptible to illness and disease in the weeks after giving birth, and also that the baby should never go without mom in the first month. Naturally, if the baby couldn't leave the house, neither should the mom. NIH*, studies show mixed feelings about this practice[9].

Now: A modern take on this is the 5-5-5 method. Five days in bed, five days on the bed, five days around the bed. This method is again meant to ensure mom is getting adequate rest and time for recovery. However, it isn't often that family is available to a new mom for an entire month. Most family members are working themselves and may have limited availability. Even if some family members are available to come and help with the baby for a few hours, in many cultures (I am thinking mainly western) family members are not always willing to do ALL the cooking and cleaning. If the new mom and dad do not have extensive funds, hiring out these services is impractical.

Additionally, getting up and moving around as soon as mom is comfortable is important as this can reduce the risks of blood clots. After getting cleared (to leave the house, or physical activity—leaving that up to you), most moms choose to make trips to her primary physician, most choose to make trips to the grocery, take walks in the park, and do cleaning around the house. Many doctors recommend waiting until the baby is a full month before taking her into crowded places such as malls, airports, or train stations.

So here, the traditional practice is much more nuanced in a modern society where most people are working and very busy in their own lives. How soon mom gets out and about will be highly dependent on her recovery and the recommendation from her primary care physician.

Hygiene

It was very intriguing to read about traditional hygiene practices and even more interesting to learn about how some of these practices are relevant today, even if modified to reflect new scientific understanding.

Then: No bathing, showers, or brushing teeth. It could even extend the previous practice to no one coming into the home for a month. It was thought that since mom is weak after child birth in her vaginal area, adding water would introduce sources of illness, inflammation, and bloating. Controlling the amount of germs introduced was important and handled by not letting extended family into the home during the postpartum period.

A mom was to use a sponge or a towel to clean herself. She would rinse her mouth with warm water and use clothes to clean her teeth. Using boiled water was recommended in order to avoid sickness.

Keep in mind that historically, most people did not have access to clean, purified water. Even today water can be a source of transmitting viruses and parasites. While a person's body at full working health is able to fight off minor viruses and germs, a person suffering from blood loss and the trauma of pregnancy and birth may not be able to do so.

Now: It is still true that hygiene after giving birth is important. Your body is still recovering and you have been through a lot physically and emotionally increasing your chances of getting sick. Bathing after birth is dependent on whether you have had a vaginal birth, c-section, or if you have stitches. If you've had a vaginal birth and no stitches, a warm bath could actually aid in recovery and help relieve pain. If you've had a c-section or needed stitches, it's recommended that you wait two weeks or longer to take a bath. Showers after twenty-four hours are fine for both vaginal births and c-sections.

It's highly important that you wash your hands before and after changing your pad and cleaning the vaginal area. There are several vaginal care kits that are sold to help with this process. You can consult with your physician on which, if any, can be used. If you have access to filtered water, using that would be better, as filtered water is free of chlorine, fluoride, heavy metals, and any potential illness.

Limiting Guests in the Home

Then: This is in line with the tradition of staying home for thirty days. This was seen as another way to prevent the spread of illness to mom and baby.

Now: This may prove helpful today as well, although one does not have to keep all visitors away. With the advent of modern medicine and hygiene and (post-pandemic) illness awareness, you can be a bit more flexible. You can require all visitors to wash their hands before handling the baby and limit visitors to close family and friends for the first few weeks. This can be determined by your and your spouse's/partner's preference and pediatrician recommendations. A tough delivery may also weigh in on who, when, and how many visitors you want in your home.

Historically, there have been a lot of myths and fears surrounding postpartum care. These stem largely from pre-modern medicine or medical conditions and the fact that, statistically, up to only one hundred years ago, one in ten women died in childbirth. However, most traditions should be celebrated as they are intended to care for mother and child in the best possible way.

These traditions bring family and friends closer to new parents as they share this time and work to be of service to one another. If you are struggling with the traditions of your parents, you can hold them in honor, while also modifying them to suit your needs and the recommendations of your physician.

CHAPTER 8

HEALING AFTER BIRTH: NATURAL REMEDIES AND TIPS

There are different ways to care for your body, depending on the kind of birth you had. Was it vaginal with little complications? Did you have tearing? Was a cesarean section performed? If so, was it scheduled or an emergency? All of these nuances can affect how you care for yourself after giving birth. Even a relatively uncomplicated (easy) birthing experience leaves behind soreness. The cervix has to heal from the baby's passage. The uterus has to contract, and all of your internal organs need to reset.

Let's get into the different areas you will need to pay attention to during your Fourth Trimester.

Perineal Care - Vaginal Birth

Perineal care after birth is essential for promoting healing, preventing infection, and ensuring overall comfort during the postpartum recovery period. After a vaginal delivery the perineal area becomes tender and vulnerable. Keeping the area clean reduces the risk of bacteria entering any wounds, which can prevent complications and support the body's natural healing process. Gentle hygiene practices, such as using a peri bottle with warm water and changing pads frequently, help soothe discomfort while minimizing irritation.

Beyond physical healing, proper perineal care supports emotional well-being by helping new parents feel more in control of their recovery. It can ease anxiety around pain or hygiene and allow for more restful moments during an already intense and transformative time. Educating birthing people about perineal care gives them the tools to care for their bodies with confidence and dignity. Something every new parent deserves.

During a vaginal birth, a few physical outcomes may occur as the baby passes through the birth canal. These include tearing, an episiotomy, or swelling of the perineal area.

- **Tears** (also known as perineal lacerations) happen naturally when the vaginal tissues stretch beyond their limit, especially in first-time births, rapid deliveries, or when the baby is large or in a challenging position. They range from minor (first-degree) to severe (fourth-degree) and may require stitches.

- An **episiotomy** is a surgical incision made in the perineum (the area between the vagina and anus) to enlarge the vaginal opening. Though less common today, it's sometimes performed in cases of fetal distress or when assisted delivery tools like forceps are used.

- Finally, **swelling** of the vaginal and perineal tissues is a common and usually temporary result of the intense pressure and fluid buildup during labor and delivery. It can be caused by prolonged pushing, the baby's position, or simply the body's natural response to trauma and exertion during birth. Each of these events is manageable and typically resolves with proper postpartum care, but knowing about them helps parents feel more prepared for the birth experience.

Postpartum bleeding, also known as **lochia,** is a normal and expected part of recovery after giving birth. It begins immediately after delivery as the body sheds the lining of the uterus, along with blood and mucus. For the first few days, the bleeding is usually heavy and bright red, similar to a heavy period, and may contain small clots. Over the following weeks, it gradually becomes lighter in color and flow, changing from red to pink, then brown, and finally yellow or white.

Postpartum bleeding usually lasts about four to six weeks but can vary from person to person. It's important to rest and avoid strenuous activity to prevent increased bleeding. However, if the bleeding suddenly becomes very heavy (soaking a pad in an hour), includes large clots, or is accompanied by dizziness or fever, it could be a sign of **postpartum hemorrhage** or infection, and medical attention should be sought immediately. Understanding what's normal and what's not can help new mothers feel more confident during recovery.

- **Witch Hazel Pads:** To alleviate discomfort and promote healing, consider using chilled witch hazel pads placed between a sanitary napkin and the perineal area. This method can provide soothing relief and reduce inflammation.
- **Herbal Support:** Incorporating herbal remedies like raspberry leaf tea may help tone and strengthen the uterus, supporting a smoother recovery. Always consult your provider before introducing herbal supplements.

- **Warm Compresses:** Applying warm heat to your abdomen or lower back can help relieve postpartum cramping (often caused by the uterus contracting back to its normal size).

- **Peri Bottles:** Use a peri bottle (a handheld squirt bottle) filled with warm water to gently cleanse the perineal area after urination or bowel movements. This prevents irritation and supports hygiene when wiping is uncomfortable.

- **Sitz Baths:** Try sitz baths (short, warm soaks for the perineal area) to reduce swelling, relieve pain, and keep the area clean. These can be done in a shallow basin or with a special sitz bath kit that fits over the toilet.

- **Rest and Elevation:** When possible, rest with your legs slightly elevated to reduce swelling and promote circulation. Using a donut-shaped cushion or soft pillow while sitting can also ease pressure on sore areas.

- **Over-the-Counter Pain Relief:** Use approved pain relief methods, like acetaminophen or ibuprofen, to manage discomfort—especially in the first few days postpartum. Always follow your provider's instructions.

Caring for a C-Section

A **Cesarean section (C-section)** is a surgical procedure used to deliver a baby through incisions made in the mother's abdomen and uterus. It may be planned ahead of time due to medical reasons—such as placenta previa, breech position, or a previous C-section—or it may become necessary during labor if complications arise, like fetal distress or stalled labor.

While C-sections are generally safe, they are still major surgeries and come with risks, including infection, increased blood loss, and longer recovery times compared to vaginal birth. Recovery usually involves a hospital stay of two to four days and several weeks of rest at home, during which lifting, driving, and strenuous activity should be limited. Some mothers may also experience emotional challenges following a C-section, especially if the procedure was unplanned, making support and education an essential part of postpartum care. Despite these challenges, C-sections are a life-saving option for many families and can be a healthy way to bring a baby into the world.

Recovery after a C-section is a gradual process that requires rest, patience, and intentional care. Since the procedure involves major abdominal surgery, your body needs time to heal—not just from childbirth, but also from the incisions in your abdomen and uterus. For the first few weeks, it's important to avoid heavy lifting (anything heavier than your baby), intense physical activity, or driving. Gentle movement, such as short walks around your home, can promote circulation and help prevent complications like blood clots. Make sure to prioritize rest whenever possible, ask for help with household tasks, and stay hydrated and nourished to support healing.

C-Section Wound Care Tips

- **Keep the incision clean and dry**: Gently wash the area with mild soap and water, then pat dry—don't scrub.
- **Avoid soaking**: Skip baths, pools, or hot tubs until your healthcare provider clears you (usually after the incision has fully healed).
- **Wear loose, breathable clothing**: This prevents irritation and helps air circulate around the incision.

- **Consider a postpartum support belt:** Some people find abdominal binders or belly bands helpful for extra support and comfort.
- **Check for signs of infection:** Contact your provider if you notice increased redness, swelling, warmth, pus, a foul smell, or if you develop a fever.
- **Support your abdomen when moving:** Hold a pillow against your belly when coughing, sneezing, or getting out of bed to reduce strain.
- **Take pain medication as prescribed:** Don't hesitate to use doctor-approved pain relief—it supports your ability to rest and heal.
- **Get help and rest:** Let others assist with daily tasks so your body can focus on recovery.

Postpartum Healing: What to Watch For

Whether you've given birth vaginally or by C-section, your body needs time, care, and attention to heal. Each recovery path has its own set of physical challenges, and it's important to recognize the signs that something may not be healing properly. Staying informed helps you know when what you're experiencing is normal—and when it might be time to reach out to your healthcare provider. With both perineal care and C-section recovery, early attention to warning signs can prevent complications and support a smoother healing journey.

Perineal Care (vaginal birth)

- Increased pain, especially after the first few days
- Foul-smelling discharge or pus from the vaginal area
- Swelling that worsens instead of improves

- Burning or difficulty urinating
- Signs of infection around stitches or tears (redness, warmth, discharge)
- Heavy bleeding (soaking a pad in an hour or passing large clots)

C-Section Care

- Redness, swelling, or warmth around the incision
- Oozing or pus coming from the incision site
- A foul odor from the incision area
- Fever or chills
- Increasing pain at the incision site instead of gradual improvement
- The incision site reopening or looking irritated
- Trouble standing or walking due to abdominal pain

CHAPTER 9

GENTLE MOVEMENT AND STRETCHING FOR RECOVERY

Engaging in gentle postpartum yoga can enhance flexibility, reduce stress, and promote overall well-being. Poses such as Cat-Cow and Child's Pose are beneficial for easing tension and supporting recovery.

For some of us, getting back into shape after giving birth is high on our list of priorities. The first thing I would like to say is:

You are beautiful right now. You are worthy right now.
You are strong right now.

Pregnancy is beautiful and arduous. It takes a lot of work for your pre-pregnancy bodies to grow and stretch and physically carry the weight of a small human being. Then one day, after nine months, approximately 273 days, the baby is born. You are no longer pregnant. Your body has been through another ordeal, that of giving birth. We all experience various levels of difficulty (and sometimes surgery) to bring life into the world.

And do we get a week off after almost a year of physical stress? Do we get to lounge around, sleep, eat nurturing meals, go to therapy, a chiropractor, a physical therapist, or gosh darn it a massage therapist?! No.

We get maybe a couple of hours, and then we are nursing or bottle-feeding. We are changing diapers and helping older siblings. We may be fortunate to have the fathers and family there, and it's still hard. Many of us do not have outside support.

And in all of this, our bodies are still physically injured. Mentally, we are processing so much change, and emotionally, we are trying … trying to be there for everyone, especially this new precious person. Getting in shape should be the last thing on our minds. Yet, for so many it is right up there with everything else that needs to happen. So please let me tell you that you are perfect right here and now with all of your imperfections.

When it comes to your body, right now, your recovery is the most important. After nine months of growing, stretching, changing, and then giving birth, your body needs time to recover and heal.

Your body may never be the same, and that's okay. You have been through a lot. You are part of your body. You have been through a lot, and you are the evidence of that.

Quite often, I find that society views the body as separate from us, as if we are operating avatars and can change skins to suit each phase and change of life. It's simply not true, and I find that concept dehumanizing. We are not in a battle against our bodies. We *are* our bodies. And we—*you*—deserve to be loved and cared for as the amazing person you are. No matter what stage or phase you are in.

Getting in shape, losing, or gaining weight is not a thing you are doing to your body. It is a thing you are doing **for** yourself. It is an act of loving kindness because you believe you deserve the best-feeling life possible. The goal is to be the healthiest version of yourself so you can show up strong in all the roles you have to fulfill.

So how can you recover, heal, and strengthen now that you are postpartum? The key is to *take it slow*.

1. Daily stretching

    Stretching is wonderful for mobility and muscle strength. It's also a great way to engage the lymphatic system and increase blood circulation, which can decrease inflammation. It helps loosen stiff joints and can help work out the kinks when you have to sit for long periods of time. Try doing simple stretches before and/or after a feeding session. Focus on arms and shoulders, neck, then lower body.

2. Walking

    Walking is another low-impact way to get healthy and strong. It increases circulation and when done outdoors, helps to connect you with nature, which has numerous benefits. I start with timing myself. Ten minutes at first, slowly increasing over time. I used to track steps versus time, but as I have entered menopause, I find that sometimes a higher step count is actually counterproductive, making me more tired and mentally drained. So I now try for thirty minutes a day, no matter the pace.

    You can try the same thing. Make a goal of twenty to thirty minutes a day. The best thing about walking is that you can absolutely take the baby with you. Push the stroller up and down the block. If there are siblings, they can enjoy a nice walk as well, maybe even before nap time or after dinner to help with sleep.

3. Light strength training

   Note that I said *light* strength training. Strength training is beneficial in that it helps you get toned and lean. Use light weights— three, five, or ten pounds—and practice curls, rows, or deadlifts. My favorite is to carry my five-pound weights for ten minutes of my daily walk. Combined with stretching and walking, strength training can really help you feel better and build endurance.

4. Swimming

   Swimming is my miracle exercise. You are weightless in the water, which helps with inflammation and reduction of gravity stress. You are getting resistance from the water so you do not need to do heavy laps in order to get a calorie burn. My favorite thing about swimming is that I can workout and NOT sweat. There is the added benefit that it is so fun and of course, the children can come along with you.

5. Low-impact workouts

   Having a routine of two to three days a week of workouts may also help to build up your energy and strength. I follow a couple channels that I feel meet my needs when it comes to working out. You can also find a group fitness class, like yoga, where you can find support in your fitness path. I do stress that if you go to a fitness class, you choose an instructor who really understands modifications and the importance of low impact. From experience, I know that an injury from working out can be a huge setback and demoralizing. You are your body's expert because you and your body are one. Do not be afraid to advocate for yourself, and you also have the right to walk away from anything that is not for you.

The goal of easing into exercise is to be healthy so that you can live a long, full life. The happier you are, the happier your family will be. If you feel you need to rest, then rest. If today you can only do a ten-minute walk, then that's fine. There is no race because there is no finish line. You will continue to grow and change, and part of that includes your body because you are your body as well.

CHAPTER 10

REST, SLEEP, AND NUTRITION

Adequate rest is vital for postpartum recovery. Aim to sleep when your baby sleeps to help your body heal. Accepting help from friends and family can allow you to focus on rest and self-care.

Consuming a balanced diet rich in protein, iron, and omega-3 fatty acids can boost energy levels and support mood stabilization. Stocking up on healthy snacks and preparing nutritious meals can make it easier to maintain a wholesome diet during this demanding time.

By integrating these holistic practices into your postpartum routine, you can foster a nurturing environment that supports both your physical recovery and overall well-being.

Understanding the Difference Between Rest and Sleep

It's easy to think of rest and sleep as the same thing—especially when you're exhausted and trying to squeeze both into the margins of your day. But they're actually quite different, and both are deeply important for your healing and well-being.

Sleep is a biological necessity. Your body needs those sleep cycles to restore, repair, and regulate everything from your hormones to your immune system. It's when your brain files memories, your tissues heal, and your nervous system gets a reset.

Rest, on the other hand, is more flexible. It's the intentional slowing down, the quiet moments in between—when you allow your body and mind to pause without needing to "do." That might mean closing your eyes for five minutes, sitting in silence, meditating, or just taking a break from stimulation.

You don't have to be asleep to be resting, and you don't have to earn rest by doing more. Both are valuable. Both are valid. In postpartum life, making space for *both* is part of caring for yourself with compassion.

In the previous chapters, we spoke of different mindfulness practices that can help you take a moment and reset in order to reduce anxiety and stress. These included journaling, meditation, listening to music and taking micro breaks. Let's look at three techniques to improve sleep.

Prioritize Rest Over Routine

In the early postpartum weeks, it's important to release expectations of structured routines—especially around sleep. The baby's circadian rhythm is still developing, and your body is healing and adjusting hormonally. Instead of focusing on strict schedules, shift your mindset to honor rest in all its forms. This means accepting short naps, lying down even if you can't sleep, and creating small windows for restorative stillness.

Sleep may come in fragmented chunks, and that's okay. Giving yourself permission to rest when your baby does—rather than catching up on chores or pushing through exhaustion—can dramatically reduce fatigue and improve your emotional resilience. It's not about "sleep when the baby sleeps" in a rigid sense, but rather, learning to identify and protect pockets of rest without guilt.

Create a Restful Sleep Environment - For You and Baby

Your environment can be a powerful tool in supporting better sleep. For both you and your baby, calming cues like dim lighting, soft white noise, and a comfortable temperature can help signal that it's time to wind down. Especially for the birthing parent, having a bedside setup that reduces how much you have to get up. For instance, a bassinet within arm's reach, water nearby, and essentials within reach can minimize disruptions.

Using aromatherapy (like lavender or chamomile), soft lighting in the evening, and limiting blue light from screens can also help regulate melatonin levels, which are often disrupted postpartum. While baby's sleep may still be inconsistent, having a peaceful space makes it easier for *you* to fall back asleep after middle-of-the-night feeds or wakings.

Lean on Support and Share the Load

One of the most effective yet underutilized ways to improve postpartum sleep is **asking for help.** Whether it's your partner, a family member, a postpartum doula, or a trusted friend, allowing others to support you in nighttime care or daytime tasks can make a world of difference. This might mean taking turns with feeds (if you're bottle-feeding or pumping), having someone hold the baby while you nap, or simply letting someone else handle meals and laundry.

Postpartum recovery isn't meant to happen in isolation. Delegating tasks so you can protect your rest is not a luxury—it's essential for physical healing, mental clarity, and emotional well-being. In cultures where "the village" steps in during the first forty days, maternal sleep outcomes are significantly better. Even small shifts in support can allow your nervous system to calm, making it easier to enter deeper, more restorative sleep cycles.

CHAPTER 11

CREATING A HEALTHY HOME ENVIRONMENT

We probably all want our homes to be as safe and healthy as possible. We go to great lengths to clean, organize, and care for our space so that our families can thrive in a comfortable environment. However, many of the everyday cleaning agents we trust to maintain a healthy home can actually introduce harmful toxins. Take Teflon cookware, for instance—long considered a kitchen staple, it's now known to release harmful chemicals when scratched or overheated. That realization led me to research healthier alternatives, and what I discovered has completely shifted how I approach home care.

Reducing exposure to "forever chemicals" by choosing natural, less toxic materials and methods is one powerful way to care for your family's health. Using glass, stoneware, stainless steel, cast iron, and copper in place of plastics can help reduce chemical absorption in the body. While you may not be able to eliminate all toxins from your life, you can take meaningful steps to minimize exposure and protect your home.

Transitioning can feel overwhelming, especially with the cost of higher-quality items such as stainless steel or cast iron. But the shift doesn't have to happen all at once—start small, build gradually, and find what works best for your lifestyle.

Homemade and Semi-Homemade Cleaners

You don't need an arsenal of store-bought sprays to keep your home fresh and clean. Making your own cleaners can be simple and effective, and ordering natural products from trusted companies like *Doterra* or *Branch Basics* can offer peace of mind.

- **All-Purpose Cleaner:** Mix white vinegar, water, and lemon for a gentle daily cleaner. Add a drop of rubbing alcohol or dish soap for extra power.
- **Bathroom Scrub:** Combine baking soda and vinegar for a fizzy, natural scrubbing agent.
- **Wood Care:** For polishing, I use Murphy's Oil once a month. Weekly, I wipe wood with a cloth and tea tree oil soap, and occasionally condition it with infused olive oil. You can also use walnut or coconut oil, infused with essential oils for a fresh scent.
- **Glass Cleaner:** A mix of water, vinegar, and a drop of lemon or rosemary essential oil leaves glass sparkling and fresh-smelling.
- **Carpet Freshener:** Mix baking soda and water with vinegar and a few drops of lemon or rosemary oil to naturally sanitize and refresh carpets.

Easy Swaps for a Healthier Home

- **Plastic to Glass:** Start with easy switches—glass spray bottles, soap dispensers, and drinking bottles. These changes add both beauty and function while reducing plastic use.

- **Cookware:** Slowly transition away from non-stick pans. Begin with one or two cast iron or stainless-steel items. Always research coatings on stoneware or ceramic pieces to ensure safety.

- **Utensils:** Wooden and stainless-steel utensils are long-lasting, easy to clean, and free from harmful additives. Use wood for scratch-prone cookware and stainless steel for everything else.

Getting Started: Small Steps Make a Big Difference

- Replace plastic water bottles with refillable glass or stainless-steel options.
- Swap plastic kitchen utensils for wooden or stainless steel.
- Try a single homemade cleaner (perhaps for mirrors or countertops) and see how you like it.
- You can choose to purchase from brands that specialize in natural home products, like Doterra or Branch Basics.

Holistic Oils for the Home

I'd love to take a moment to share two of my favorite oils that have become staples in our home: olive oil and castor oil. These versatile oils support a holistic lifestyle and offer surprising benefits.

Olive Oil

Cooking:

Extra virgin olive oil (EVOO) is rich in monounsaturated fatty acids (MUFAs), which support heart and brain health by balancing cholesterol. It's best consumed at room temperature—drizzled over salads, vegetables, or bread. EVOO can also be added to herbal pestos. Some traditions suggest taking one to two teaspoons on an empty stomach in the morning to boost wellness.

Skin Care:

Olive oil contains antioxidants such as Vitamin E that reduce inflammation and soothe skin conditions like eczema. Apply a small amount directly or mix with your regular moisturizer to support healthy, glowing skin.

Oral Care:

Oil pulling with olive oil (swishing one to two tablespoons for up to twenty minutes and then spitting it out) can help remove toxins and support oral hygiene.

Polishing:

Olive oil can be used on wood, leather, or stainless steel to buff and shine. Add essential oils like lemon or rosemary for an antibacterial and aromatic finish.

Caution:

Olive oil is rich and thick—use it in small amounts or dilute it to avoid clogged pores. It's not a cleaner on its own, but it's an amazing compliment to natural cleaning and care practices.

Castor Oil

Skin:

Packed with vitamin E, omega-6 and 9, and ricinoleic acid, castor oil deeply hydrates and can support healing for conditions like eczema and minor skin imperfections. Mix with a carrier oil like coconut or olive oil for gentler application.

Medicinal & Immunity:

Its antimicrobial and anti-inflammatory properties make castor oil a great option for joint pain, immunity support, and even wound care. Swishing small amounts in the mouth or applying to feet may support detoxification.

Arthritis Relief:

Apply to sore joints with a warm cloth to ease swelling and improve mobility. Daily use offers the best results.

Constipation:

FDA-approved for short-term relief, castor oil can be ingested—but only occasionally and in very small doses. Some also use it topically over the abdomen, though this practice is more traditional than it is medically confirmed.

Baby Care:

Use with caution! Never give castor oil internally to infants, and always consult a pediatrician before topical use. If used, dilute it well with a mild carrier oil.

Cautions:

Avoid castor oil during pregnancy (as it can stimulate contractions), and limit internal use. Always test for allergies first by applying a small amount to the skin.

Knowing how to use the ingredients and tools already in your home empowers you to live a safer, more intentional life. Whether you're switching to glassware, mixing up a new cleaning solution, or tapping into ancient remedies, small shifts can make a big impact.

NATURE IMMERSION

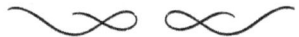

STEP TWO - CONNECT

Definition 1) Bring together or into contact so that a real or notional link is established. Join together to provide access and communication. Link to a power or water supply.

Connecting with nature is more than just being outside. It's about opening yourself as a conduit for healing and communication. It's a way of acknowledging that you are part of something vast, ancient, and in many ways, unknowable. Yet, when you allow yourself to truly connect, you begin to understand both nature and yourself in a deeply personal way.

Connection to self, to nature, and to others is vital for mental health. It mirrors the body's circulatory system, creating a continuous flow of energy, belonging, and well-being. When you disconnect, when you isolate and disengage, that flow is disrupted, leaving us feeling drained, stagnant, and depleted.

As new mothers, whether caring for one child or several, it's easy to lose that sense of connection. Our days revolve around feeding schedules, sleep routines, and household tasks, and we may feel our vital energy slowing, or even stopping altogether. This exhaustion (both physical and mental) can make postpartum recovery even more challenging.

But even amidst these challenges, you can still foster connection. Nature, in particular, offers a direct link to something greater than ourselves, providing immediate comfort and renewal. When you step outside, even briefly, you may find the healing, grounding, and connection needed to sustain your well-being. This simple act re-energizes you, restoring that flow and stimulating you toward whatever action you need in that moment.

Walking Nature Reflection and Activity

Go for a walk (you can take the baby/children with you), but if possible, try to go alone. Start by walking at an easy pace for five to ten minutes, allowing yourself to settle into the rhythm of movement. Tune into the sensations around you, the feeling of the wind on your skin, the warmth of the sun, or the coolness of light rain. Listen to the sounds that surround you: the rustling of leaves, the chirping of birds, the distant bark of a dog. Notice how the sounds shift depending on your location, such as a park, a wooded trail, or your neighborhood. Pay attention to how these sensory experiences make you feel.

Just as we nurture our children, we must also remember to nurture ourselves. While walking one morning, during a particularly hard time in my life, I saw a walnut husk. Something about it called to me, so I picked it up and turned it over. The inside was shaped like a heart. It struck me that even though I was going through it, I was being watched over. It reminded me that if I look for it, I will find love and care all around me. It gave me strength. I still have that husk on my desk. I look at it from time to time, and it always brings me back to that moment of love and connection.

As you walk, look for a treasure that speaks to you. This practice invites a sense of childlike wonder—after all, children love to collect treasures from their walks. Your small treasure can be a rock, a stick, a leaf, or a feather. Hold it in your hands, or if it's a tree, place your open palm against the bark. Take a deep breath, and notice the first thought or feeling that comes to mind. If nothing stands out, that's okay. Sometimes, the connection isn't immediately obvious. Choose something anyway.

When you bring it home, take a moment to reflect on why it caught your attention and how it makes you feel. Let it serve as a small reminder of your connection to nature and yourself.

Alternative

You can do this activity in your yard, on your balcony, or even by a window. You may notice a leaf, a feather, or a pebble—choose one of these objects, and use it as part of your exercise. If no physical object is available, you can connect with the sky, the moon, or the sun instead.

LIIT Exercise: Toe to Ceiling Reaches

This is a great full-body exercise that is low-impact and easily adjustable to increase intensity. Start by standing with your feet hip-width apart. Raise your arms straight overhead, then reach down to touch the ground, bending your knees as needed. Straighten back up, lifting your arms toward the ceiling once more. Repeat this movement ten times, then rest for twenty seconds.

If you're feeling up to it, complete two or three sets. You can begin at a slow, controlled pace and gradually increase speed for a more intense workout, or maintain a steady pace and add more repetitions over time.

As always, listen to your body and be mindful as you rebuild your strength.

To modify this exercise, try doing it seated. Reach toward the ground. Extend your arms toward the ceiling, maintaining a steady rhythm. This adjustment allows you to engage in movement while honoring your body's needs.

Mindfulness Breath Practice: Alternate Nostril Breathing

Sit in a comfortable position and relax your shoulders. Place your thumb on the side of one nostril and gently close it. Breathe in through the open nostril. Switch by lifting your thumb and using your index finger to push down on the other nostril. Breathe out through the open nostril. Do this for one minute. This breathing exercise will help reduce stress and increase lung capacity, aiding in increased endurance. It can also help to improve the connection between the heart and lungs, helping them work together in a more fluid manner.

Dietary Focus: Stews

Stews, like soups, are a comforting and nourishing meal that can be easily packed with nutrient-dense vegetables, proteins, and wholesome carbohydrates. They provide warmth and sustenance without being too heavy. This makes them gentle on digestion, especially important during postpartum recovery. Stews are also ideal for meal prepping and storing, allowing you to have a ready-to-eat, nourishing option on hand.

One of my favorite healing stews is chicken stew. It's rich in protein and essential nutrients. When made with ingredients like carrots, onions, garlic, and herbs, it becomes a rich source of vitamins A, K, and D, as well as antioxidants that support immunity, reduce inflammation, and promote overall well-being.

Journal Questions

Food, for many of us, has emotional and traditional ties. Think of your favorite stew (if you have one). What thoughts, feelings, memories, or emotions does it call to mind? If you could meal prep stews, what would you make? How do you feel about meal prepping?

Step Two - Connect

Describe the object you found on your walk. What emotions does it evoke? As you held it or gazed at it from a distance, what thoughts or memories surfaced?

Think back to my story about finding the walnut hull and how it helped me feel loved and cared for. In what ways does your object reflect your journey or aspects of yourself? What message does your found treasure hold for you?

Artist Within ~ Infinite Connection

Create a visual representation of your connection to nature and the world around you. Consider how energy flows through you, much like the circulatory system, linking you to the earth, the sky, and the life surrounding you. Use colors, textures, and movement to express the sensation of belonging, renewal, and healing. Your piece can be abstract or symbolic—perhaps a tree with roots extending into the swirling cosmos, or a figure intertwined with the elements.

SECTION III

Navigating Relationships

CHAPTER 12

THERE IS LOVE ENOUGH FOR ALL

Navigating relationships during the postpartum period is essential for fostering a supportive environment that benefits both you and your newborn. This chapter provides strategies to enhance communication with your partner, set healthy boundaries with family and friends, and build a community that supports your new role as a mother.

Older Children

Building strong relationships between older siblings and a newborn starts with creating a sense of inclusion and importance for the older child. It's essential to acknowledge their feelings, offer reassurance, and give them age-appropriate ways to participate in caring for the baby. Simple tasks, such as fetching a diaper, singing to the baby, or helping during bath time, can foster a sense of responsibility and pride.

Setting aside one-on-one time with the older sibling also helps maintain their emotional connection with parents, reducing feelings of jealousy or displacement. Celebrating their new role as a big brother or sister, while also validating the challenges, lays the foundation for a bond rooted in love, trust, and shared family identity.

Being a parent is challenging in many ways. I could write an entire book on the challenges of parenthood. One challenging question for postpartum mothers and parents of siblings is, "How do we divide our time between the children?"

If you have older children, it can be challenging to balance the needs of your baby with those of your other child(ren). Integrating a new infant into the family successfully requires that everyone feels accepted and loved equally.

Babies have specific needs that must be met for them to thrive physically. These needs should not be neglected. So how can you manage to give each child the attention they need?

Plan Ahead

Even if it's five minutes, plan some time each day with each child. What you do during this time will vary depending on the age of your child and their interests. For instance, some older children may just need time to talk or sit with you quietly. Others may enjoy building a LEGO tower or doing a creative activity such as coloring. Some may want you to read a book with them.

Whatever you choose, make sure they know that this time with them is sacred. This time, as much as possible, should not be interrupted by phone calls, TV, social media, etc. This is one-on-one time with only them, doing something that brings you both joy.

Choose Your Timing Carefully

This may require some forethought and paying attention to your routine and the new baby's routine. If you know the baby sleeps from 1 to 3 p.m. every day, you may devote thirty minutes of this nap time to spend time with your older child(ren). If you and your older child are up while the baby sleeps in, this is a great way to share quality time together.

You can even say something like, "Brian is asleep for another twenty minutes. What should we do, just the two of us, before we get hugs from baby brother?" This keeps it fun and shows that you want to spend time with both of them. It is not one against the other. Both can be loved individually.

Communicate

Even younger children benefit greatly from clear, open, and honest communication. Be clear in saying what tasks need to be accomplished. You may need to work, clean, or make meals. However, for these thirty, twenty, or fifteen minutes, etc., you are theirs alone. This will help to establish healthy boundaries for you and your child. It will also model time management skills and teach them how to prioritize from an early age.

Be Flexible

No matter how much you plan, life happens. The nap that used to last from 1:00 to 3:00 is now from 2:00 to 3:00, and the project that your boss wanted two weeks from now, well … they want it this week. Things happen, so flexibility is key. Again, clear, open communication with your older children will help. Instead of calling your one-on-one time a wash, you can shorten it and make up for it another day or even later in the day. The key is to have some quality time each day. This will instill in your child that they are important. *No Matter What* life throws at you, you will always prioritize them.

Parenting multiple children is hard. There is no way around it. However, simple adjustments can be made, and with a little planning and a lot of patience, you can be confident that you will give each child love and attention.

Spouse/Partner

Welcoming a newborn into the family is a life-changing experience that can bring joy and connection, but it also challenges the dynamics of a couple's relationship. The physical and emotional demands of caring for a baby—especially the lack of sleep, feeding schedules, and recovery from birth— can leave little room for quality time or meaningful communication between partners.

It's important to acknowledge that your relationship may feel different during this season and that this shift is normal. Open, compassionate communication becomes the anchor. Sharing how you're each feeling, checking in regularly, and being honest about your needs creates space for emotional support and reduces misunderstandings.

Maintaining connection doesn't require grand gestures. Small acts of kindness, simple affirmations, and even a few minutes of undistracted time together can nurture your bond. Consider scheduling brief "couple check-ins" or creating small routines like a shared cup of tea after the baby is asleep. Show appreciation for each other's contributions, whether it's changing diapers, managing household tasks, or offering a supportive word. Remember, you are a team. Nurturing your relationship during this time not only strengthens your partnership but also models a healthy connection for your growing family.

When one partner is physically distant due to work, military service, or other obligations, welcoming a newborn can feel especially isolating for the parent at home. The demands of newborn care combined with postpartum recovery can intensify feelings of loneliness, overwhelm, and even resentment. For the long-distance partner, there may be feelings of helplessness or guilt.

Maintaining connection during this time requires intentionality and creativity. Regular check-ins via video calls, shared photo albums, or even recording short voice notes for each other can help bridge the emotional gap. Talking about daily wins, hard moments, and simply being present—even virtually—helps reinforce the bond and reminds both partners they're in this together, even when apart.

When postpartum mental health challenges are part of the picture, such as anxiety, depression, or trauma recovery, it's crucial to approach the relationship with empathy and patience. Communication may be more vulnerable or strained, and emotions can feel overwhelming. Normalize the experience and seek support as a team, whether through counseling, support groups, or professional help. The partner not experiencing the mental health challenges can offer presence, nonjudgmental listening, and validation rather than solutions.

It's also important to remember to care for one another. Both parents deserve support and space to express their needs. By prioritizing compassion, shared responsibility, and emotional honesty, couples can strengthen their relationship even during one of life's most tender and trying transitions.

Enhancing Partner Communication
Effective communication with your partner is vital as you both adjust to the changes that come with parenthood.

- **Practice Empathy and Understanding:** Acknowledge each other's experiences and feelings. Being open and honest fosters mutual support.

- **Schedule Regular Check-Ins:** Set aside time to discuss feelings, responsibilities, and any concerns. This ensures both partners are heard and can collaboratively address issues.

- **Use "I" Statements:** Express emotions without assigning blame to promote constructive conversations.

By prioritizing open communication, you can strengthen your partnership and navigate the challenges of new parenthood together.

Friendships

Keeping up with a newborn's schedule is tough. If there are older children at home, it makes things a bit more complicated. Cooking, cleaning, sleep training, school schedules ... The first couple of months can go by in a blur. Finding time to relax is a chore in and of itself. Life is busy. Once you have children, it becomes busier.

Then a call comes in. It's Janice, and she wants you to come hang out with the girls. Frank invites your other half over for beer, pizza, and a boxing match on the big screen. You have finally found a rhythm, a routine. It's not the time to break that rhythm, so you decline, "next time." Yet, next time may not be good either. The baby might be sick, or some other child-related event might happen.

A funny thing can happen when we become parents. We seem not to have time for friends. This is especially true if we are the first among our friends to do so. Late nights out are no longer a thing, and there is precious little time to spend on entertainment that does not include the children. Time with friends lessens. In some cases, we can become so estranged from friends that we, in effect, lose their valuable support at a time we greatly need it.

Having children makes them the priority. There is no arguing with that. However, it's good to remember that your ability to maintain healthy relationships in and out of the home is vital to your mental health and an important model for your children. While keeping up with friendships takes time and effort, you have options!

Something for Everyone

Find outings that can be enjoyed by all. While nights out on the dance floor or living it up at the sports bar may be out for a while, you can still have fun and spend quality time with your friends. Activities such as hiking or a stroll in the park are great options. Pack a picnic and beverages, or have an early dinner at a venue that accommodates both adults and children. Several shopping areas have restaurants and some green space (small park-like areas with grass or turf) for families to lounge. It may take a little research, but you can definitely find places that allow you to have fun and bring the children along.

Stay In

Conversely, staying home might be a better option. Sure, there may be laundry or toys scattered about. If your friends are true, they will not care! Invite them over for brunch or even dinner. Staying home gives you a level of situational control that cannot be had anywhere else. You know your home is childproof. You know what your child can and cannot touch.

Plus, you can skip the effort of packing the safari-sized bags often needed when leaving home with kids. Have a movie night, game night, cards, and wine. The list is endless. You can excuse yourself when it's time to put the little ones to sleep or plan your event around the children's sleep schedules.

Include Your Friends in Your Daily Life
There are so many celebratory milestones in our children's lives—the baby rolled over, their first tooth, and their first time sleeping through the night, etc. Even older children have milestones and events—the school play or festival, and social events for clubs. These are things that can go overlooked as ways to include friends. Why not occasionally invite them? They may not take you up on it. Maybe they will. Most importantly, this shows them that you value their presence in your life and you want to share what's important to you with them.

Communicate, Communicate, Communicate
To *have* great friends, one must *be* a great friend. It seems obvious, but **call** your friends. Take time to ask about how they are doing. Listen. Sure, you may realize that after having children, the word *tired* means something different to you. This does not invalidate that they also get tired, stressed out, and demoralized.

Having their friend hear them out can make all the difference. The more you listen, the more readily they will also listen when you need to unload. At the end of the day, it's the emotional bonding from sincere communication that helps make friendships strong and long-lasting.

Accept Change
Unfortunately, some friendships may not survive after you become parents. People grow and change, and sometimes you are in different places on your journeys. This may mean that some friendships take a back seat or exit your life altogether.

This isn't necessarily a negative thing. It's just that your life has changed; you have different schedules, routines, and responsibilities. This may not be accommodating to all people, and that's okay. Take time to mourn your loss, but know that all things, even friendships, have their time and place. New friendships will be made. There is always the hope of reconnecting later in life when maybe your life and theirs are no longer so different.

More Ideas for Family and Friends
Movies

Plays

Concerts

Museums

Farmer's markets

Zoos

Family
Relatives and extended family can be a valuable source of support during the newborn stage, offering help with meals, chores, or even holding the baby so parents can rest. However, navigating these relationships can be complex, especially when opinions, boundaries, or parenting styles differ. New parents need to communicate clearly about the kind of support they need and what they don't.

Setting gentle but firm boundaries around visiting hours, baby care preferences, or the need for quiet time can reduce stress and protect the healing and bonding process. Most family members want to help; they just need guidance on how to do so in ways that truly support the parents and baby.

At the same time, this is also an opportunity to build stronger intergenerational connections. Grandparents, aunts, uncles, and cousins may feel excited to be part of the baby's life, and including them in small, meaningful ways like reading to the baby, preparing a favorite family dish, or sharing stories can create lasting bonds. It's okay if relationships shift during this time. New parenthood often reshapes family dynamics, and approaching these changes with openness and mutual respect can help families grow closer while honoring the needs of the new family unit.

Setting Boundaries

Establishing clear boundaries is crucial to protect your family's well-being during this transitional period.

- Define Your Needs: Reflect on what you and your partner require regarding visits, assistance, and personal space. Being clear with yourselves helps in communicating effectively with others.

- Communicate Expectations Early: Discuss your postpartum plans with family and friends before the baby arrives. This proactive approach sets clear expectations and reduces potential misunderstandings.

- Be Firm Yet Compassionate: It's acceptable to decline requests or offers that don't align with your needs. Express gratitude for their concern while emphasizing your current priorities.

Remember, setting boundaries isn't about distancing loved ones but creating a nurturing environment for your immediate family.

Work Relationships

Navigating work relationships after having a new baby involves balancing professional responsibilities with the new demands of parenthood. Whether you're returning to work after leave or working while caring for your baby, communication is key. It helps to set realistic expectations with supervisors and colleagues, especially when flexibility is needed for childcare, feeding schedules, or medical appointments.

Being transparent (within your comfort level) about your current capacity can foster understanding and support. Many employers and coworkers are more accommodating than we expect, especially when we proactively communicate needs and boundaries.

At the same time, maintaining professional relationships while adjusting to parenthood requires self-compassion. You may not be able to perform at your previous pace right away, and that's okay. Lean into resources like employee assistance programs, supportive colleagues, or parent networks within your organization if available.

Sharing small updates, expressing appreciation, and staying engaged - when possible - can keep you connected to your professional community without adding pressure. Remember, building a sustainable work-life rhythm takes time, and it's okay to prioritize your well-being and your family as you find your footing.

NATURE IMMERSION

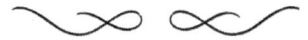

STEP THREE - ACCEPT

*Definition 1) Consent to receive (a thing offered)
2) Believe or come to recognize (an opinion,
explanation, etc.) as valid or correct*

Accept. Accepting. Acceptance. These three words can feel like the hardest part of recovery. You may feel as if you have given up your body to carry and nurture life. You have sacrificed your time, energy, and mental clarity. You have endured pain: physical, emotional, and even spiritual. You may have questioned your ability to be the kind of parent you envisioned.

You may have chosen to stay home, putting your career on pause, while others you know have returned to work, feeling judged or as if they are no longer seen as capable. No matter your path, you have changed forever. And accepting that change can be incredibly difficult.

The postpartum period can be a confusing space, filled with longing to move past the weight gain, the emotional highs and lows, the exhaustion, the sleepless nights. Everything. Yet, just like pregnancy, postpartum must run its course. Healing takes time. Mind, body, and spirit all need care in their own way. Rather than forcing acceptance all at once, try focusing on just one aspect at a time.

If you're struggling with body image, remind yourself: "This is just for this moment in time. I am proud of my body and all it has endured. I honor the sacrifice it made to bring life into this world. Today, I choose to love my body just as it is." If you're facing the weight of the baby blues, remind yourself: "I feel this way in this moment, but I know feelings can change. I am proud of my mind for all it has endured to keep me and my baby safe. I have choices, I have support, and I have the right to seek help when I need it."

To accept yourself in this vulnerable stage is an act of love. It is giving yourself permission to heal, to be patient, and to embrace the journey one step at a time.

Walking Nature Reflection

As you walk, take a moment to observe the trees and plants around you. Look specifically for those that have weathered storms, the ones that stand apart from their tall, straight counterparts. A wind-twisted cedar, with its curves, knots, and uniquely shaped branches, holds a beauty all its own. A small plant pushing through the cracks of a sidewalk may never grow into a lush bush, but its resilience makes it more powerful than those that wither under the same conditions.

As you move through nature, try to connect with one tree, plant, or natural object that carries imperfections. Notice its shape, its texture, its story. If you feel drawn to it, place your hand on its bark or take a photo to reflect on later. Let it be a reminder that strength and beauty are not always found in perfection—but in endurance, adaptation, and growth.

LIIT Exercise: Side Twists

Sit on a pillow or exercise mat with your knees bent and heels planted firmly on the ground, about shoulder-width apart. Lean back slightly, only as far as feels comfortable, while engaging your core. From this position, twist your torso side to side, aiming for a total of twenty twists. You can keep your arms in a boxing position, fists clenched close to your body or elbows out, fingertips facing toward each other or fully outstretched, whatever feels more comfortable or more challenging. Complete two sets of twenty, focusing on controlled movement and steady breathing.

Mindfulness Breath Practice: 4-7-8 Technique

Find a place to sit comfortably. Breathe in through your nose to the count of four. Hold your breath to the count of seven. Exhale to the count of eight. Repeat this for a minute or two. Of course, feel free to perform this practice longer if you like.

This technique can help you reduce anxiety when it comes on suddenly. It can help regulate food cravings, improve sleep, and help with strong emotions like anger or fear. By reducing the underlying cause of these habits (stress and anxiety), the 4-7-8 technique helps to regulate emotion, which, in turn, can help you regulate emotional eating.

Alternative

Look out of your window or go to a place just outside your home, look for a weather-worn tree, a plant pushing through the concrete, or other growing life that seems to have overcome obstacles to exist on this plane.

If needed, you can modify the activities to suit your space and comfort level. Try them seated or standing in your yard, on a patio or balcony, or even indoors by a window. If you'd like to walk but can't go outside, pacing or stepping in place is a great alternative. You'd be surprised how quickly your step count adds up or how effectively you can reach a healthy heart rate, just by marching in place.

Here is another way to modify twists: Sit upright with legs crossed, then twist side to side with your arms extended or bent.

Dietary Focus: Fruit, Yogurt, and Oatmeal

Fruit, yogurt, and oatmeal are a nutrient-rich trio that provides essential nourishment—especially in the postpartum period and beyond. Fruits supply vital vitamins, antioxidants, and natural sugars for sustained energy. Yogurt delivers probiotics to support gut health and digestion while offering a good source of protein and calcium. Calcium is a much-needed vitamin, as women are at a higher risk of osteoporosis after childbirth. Oatmeal is packed with fiber, promoting healthy digestion and stable blood sugar levels.

For those who are lactose intolerant, there are several useful alternatives, including an oat-based yogurt. Check in your local grocery store for a brand that suits your needs. Together, these foods create a balanced, wholesome meal that supports recovery, boosts energy, and enhances overall well-being, all while being simple, satisfying, and easy to incorporate into your daily routine.

Journal Questions

What types of food do you associate with happiness and feelings of pleasure? Why?

Reflect on a weather-worn tree or resilient plant you connected with on your walk or in-home reflection practice. How does its perseverance mirror your own experiences? How does imperfection shape both strength and beauty?

Step Three - Accept

Consider the challenges you've overcome, the support you've had, or lack thereof. Write about how you managed this time of your life. How has this change shaped you?

Artist Within ~ Metamorphosis

Depict your personal transformation through symbolism, like a butterfly emerging, a tree shedding leaves, or a river carving its way through the landscape.

SECTION IV

Practical Parenting Tips

CHAPTER 13

NEWBORN CARE

Caring for a newborn is a rewarding yet challenging journey. Implementing practical strategies can help you navigate this period with confidence and ease. This chapter offers holistic approaches to support you in understanding your baby's needs while maintaining your well-being.

Understanding Newborn Sleep Patterns

Newborns have irregular sleep cycles, often waking every two to three hours for feeding. Recognizing this as a normal phase can alleviate stress. **To manage irregular sleep:**

- **Create a Calming Bedtime Routine.** Engage in soothing activities like gentle rocking or soft singing to signal bedtime.
- **Observe Sleep Cues.** Learn to identify signs of sleepiness, such as eye rubbing or fussiness, to put your baby to sleep before overtiredness sets in. This can be tricky, as sometimes tiredness cues and crying can seem like hunger cues. Don't worry. This happens to even the most seasoned child care specialist. Over time, you will learn their cues. If you are not sure and it is earlier than you would normally feed them, try a pacifier and rocking or

soothing them to sleep first. If they still seem hungry, you can try to feed them next.

- **Prioritize Safe Sleep Practices.** Always place your baby on their back in a crib with a firm mattress and no loose bedding to reduce the risk of Sudden Infant Death Syndrome (SIDS). There should be no fluffy blankets, bumpers, or even sheepskin pads in the crib or bassinet. Swaddle baby and dress her in footie onesies to keep warm. Sleep is a challenge for many infants. As their body adjusts to a new rhythm and to feeding externally (outside the womb), they will wake to eat and eliminate. As the days and weeks progress and they become more aware of their surroundings, they will awaken for longer periods. This will include the nighttime. Establishing a healthy bedtime is part consistency and part timing.

Understanding and adapting to your baby's sleep needs fosters better rest for both of you.

Feeding Support: Breastfeeding, Pumping, and Bottle Feeding

Feeding is a central aspect of newborn care. Whether you choose breastfeeding, pumping, or formula feeding, consider the following:

- **Seek Professional Guidance.** Consult a lactation consultant or healthcare provider for personalized advice and to address any challenges. A postpartum doula can help support you by setting up your physical environment, creating a calming setting for the baby, and guiding you through the process.

- **Establish a Comfortable Feeding Environment.** Choose a quiet, comfortable spot to make feeding sessions more relaxing. Try to take time to nurse the baby in a quiet place for just the two of you. It can be tempting to nurse on the go (so to speak) while dealing with older children. However, it's good to try and do a couple feedings alone so that you and baby have a chance to bond. This will also help you and baby destress and can aid in better digestion. Try breastfeeding while laying on your side. It helps compress and narrow the nipple and may help with latching.

- **Stay Hydrated and Nourished.** Maintain your health to support milk production and overall energy levels.

- **Air-dry nipples after breastfeeding.** To help with sore nipples, allow them to air dry after feeding the baby. You may also apply shea butter or coconut oil to moisturize. You can also apply a little of your breastmilk. One-hundred percent cotton t-shirts and bras will help lessen soreness as cotton is a softer and natural material. Keep a little basket of snacks while breastfeeding the baby. This will help you to increase your milk production and prevent uncomfortable hunger while nursing. While it takes two hundred fifty to three hundred extra calories to grow a baby, it takes an extra five-hundred calories to produce milk and feed your precious little one.

Remember, the best feeding method is one that ensures your baby is nourished and you are comfortable with the process.

Creating Soothing Routines for Baby (and You)

Consistent routines provide security for your baby and can simplify your day. We all know sleep is important for everyone.

This includes children and infants. The first days home can feel like a sleep deprivation marathon with baby feeding every one-and-a-half to two hours (more for cluster feeders). When and how long your newborn sleeps is a topic for conversation.

Recently, there has been a large focus on sleep training for infants with a few different methods of doing so. Some methods require very strict scheduling on the part of the parent to obtain optimal sleep at night for the child. While sleep is important, there are those who believe sleep training is non-traditional and not natural for the infant.

Traditionally, parents did not sleep train their babies. In the 18th century and earlier, babies slept whenever. It did not matter if there was a lot of noise or it was daylight outside. Many mothers "wore" their babies while they went about their daily work, and the child would drift between feeding, wakefulness, and sleep. At night, infants often slept in the same bed as their parents. The rationale was that babies sleep better when they feel secure.

Of course, we are no longer in the 18th century. While sleep training seems to be a modern phenomenon, it was first brought into thought in 1894 by Dr. Luther Emmett Holt. In his book, *The Care and Feeding of Children.* His writing encourages proper feeding during the day so that the baby can sleep at night. He also seems to have pioneered the idea that babies should always sleep in a separate bed from parents to avoid being smothered.[10]

While I do not agree with his limited physical contact approach and his strict routine, I do feel that sleep training can be helpful. When done in a way that suits the whole family's needs and is adapted to the needs of your baby, it can be a useful method that adds to the daily success of family life.

So, how do you sleep train an infant?

There are several methods, and the two I find families like the most are Mom's on Call and Taking Cara Baby. Since these are well-known sources and both have books explaining in detail how to perform their method, I will only paraphrase here.

The Mom's on Call method requires a strict adherence to feeding, napping, and bedtime routine schedules. Both Mom's On Call and Taking Cara Baby encourage swaddling and the use of noise machines and darkness at night and light during the day to help acclimate the baby to a daytime wakefulness and nighttime sleepiness schedule.

However, not everyone can adhere to strict schedules. Some families travel. Others have jobs that require time away from home. Community and religious obligations may call them to be at gatherings on certain evenings of the week. Setting up an infant on a strict sleeping schedule only to interrupt it, will be counterproductive and cause further confusion at bedtime.

What are the basic ways to promote healthy sleep routines?

1. **Encourage wakeful eating.** Try to keep the baby awake while feeding. You can gently lift and lower the baby's arms and move her legs to try and energize her to wakefulness. Change the baby's diaper before feeding, and keep the baby in just a diaper for this time. This way, she does not get too warm and cozy while feeding. This gives the added benefit of having skin-to-skin time while feeding. This will be difficult in the first couple of weeks, but maintain this routine as it will greatly improve nighttime sleeping over time.

2. **Keep daytime light and nighttime dark.** Keep lights low and/or off in the area where the baby will be sleeping at night. Over time, this will make the connection that nighttime is for sleeping. Conversely, keep areas bright and well-lit during the day. Even if the baby is sleeping during the day, which he will be at first, he will come to learn that daytime is for play. As babies get older and they're having longer wake times and more structured naps, you can let them sleep in a darker room.

3. **Try the swaddle method.** Babies enjoy feeling protected and safe while asleep. Swaddling may help promote this feeling, allowing them to sleep better. You can also swaddle only at night and allow them free range during the day to further encourage longer sleep times during the evening hours.

4. **Have a bedtime routine.** It is never too early to read to baby. You can establish a one- or two-book routine. One idea is to feed, wipe down with a warm cloth or a bath, dress in a fresh diaper and pjs. Then, read your books and put baby down. The idea is to try and keep feeding separate from falling asleep *if you can*. You can follow your bedtime routine even if you cannot adhere to a strict schedule. So make it something that you can take on the go or do once you get home. The added benefit is the bonding that develops between parent and child during these gentle moments. If a child needs to feel safe so they can sleep (and we all do), then this is a sure way to instill that sense of safety, love, and security.

5. **Noise maker.** These devices produce white noise and further help to distinguish sleep time from awake time and also help to block out other intrusive sounds. White

noise mimics the sounds she heard while nestled in the womb. For best results, use a setting that produces continuous low monotone sounds. Start the "music" during your sleepy time routine, and over time, this will signal to your little one that now it's time to sleep.

6. **Be Flexible!** Not all of these methods will work for you or your values around proper sleep time. Feel free to combine these methods. There is no wrong way, as long as you and baby are safe and comfortable during sleep periods.

Getting the baby to sleep through the night takes time. So do not feel disappointed if it doesn't go perfectly at first. And as she grows, she will have times of sleeplessness. So think of this not as a straight road but a road with hills. There will be ups and downs, so always be patient with the baby and yourself.

In the resources section, you will find a reference to a reputable source for information of safeR co-sleeping. Always note that the recommendation from the American Pediatric Association is to have baby sleep separately in a crib or bassinet.

CHAPTER 14

BALANCING RESPONSIBILITIES AND SELF-CARE

Before we head into the next section, I want to pause and remind you of something essential: Your well-being matters just as much as your baby's. You've brought new life into the world, and while it's natural to turn your attention fully to your newborn, your healing, your rest, and your emotional health are vital too. You cannot pour from an empty cup. Postpartum self-care isn't selfish, it's necessary.

Below are some gentle yet powerful reminders to help you center yourself during this tender and transformative time.

Accept Help Without Guilt

Let's start here, because this is often the hardest one. Asking for or accepting help can feel uncomfortable. You might think, *"I should be able to do this on my own,"* or worry about being a burden. But here's the truth: **You were never meant to parent in isolation.**

In many traditional cultures, the postpartum period is a time when the entire community steps in to care for the new parent.

Meals are prepared, laundry is done, and the mother is given space to rest, heal, and bond with her baby. In our modern, often individualistic society, this support has faded but that doesn't mean you have to do everything alone.

Let your loved ones help. If someone offers to bring a meal, say yes. If your best friend wants to take the baby for a walk so you can nap or shower, let them. Create a "yes list" ahead of time. Small tasks others can easily do that lighten your load, like folding laundry, making a grocery run, or washing bottles. Accepting help not only supports your physical recovery, but it also fosters connection, which is just as crucial for emotional well-being.

Set Realistic Expectations for Yourself and Others

One of the most common sources of stress in early postpartum life comes from trying to do too much, too soon. Whether it's the pressure to keep the house tidy, cook every meal from scratch, or maintain social obligations, it's easy to feel overwhelmed by all the "shoulds."

Let this be your permission slip: **You do not have to be everything to everyone.**

This is a season of slowing down, of simplifying. It's okay if your home is a little messy. It's okay if you wear the same cozy robe three days in a row. It's okay if your only accomplishments today were feeding your baby and brushing your teeth.

Instead of a long to-do list, choose *one or two gentle priorities* each day. That might mean taking a short walk, journaling for ten minutes, or simply drinking water and sitting outside in the sunshine. Give yourself grace. You are not falling behind—you are deep in the sacred work of becoming.

Schedule Personal Time (Yes, Even Now)

It might sound counterintuitive or even impossible, but taking time for yourself in small, intentional ways can replenish you in profound ways. You don't need hours of solitude or a weekend getaway to recharge (though if you have access to that, amazing!)

Start with just five or ten minutes. Time to read a few pages of a book you love. Time to stretch or move your body gently. Time to write down a thought, a feeling, a memory. Time to breathe deeply with your eyes closed and remember who *you* are beyond the diapers, the feeding schedules, and the sleep-deprived nights.

Scheduling personal time isn't about stepping away from your baby, it's about reconnecting with yourself. When you tend to your own emotional and physical needs, you become more present, patient, and attuned. Not just for your baby, but for yourself and everyone around you.

Redefine What Self-Care Means

In our culture, self-care is often sold as bubble baths and spa days. While those things are lovely, true postpartum self-care is deeper. Nourishing your nervous system, protecting your peace, and honoring your healing.

It might mean saying "no" to visitors if you're feeling overwhelmed. It might mean eating warm, nutrient-dense meals that support hormonal balance and tissue repair. It might mean turning off your phone to avoid the flood of comparison and noise. It might mean crying and letting yourself feel everything you've been holding in.

Real self-care is about self-honoring and listening to what your body, heart, and spirit need each day and responding with compassion, not criticism.

Balance Giving with Receiving

As a new parent, you are in constant giving mode. You give your time, your body, your sleep, your attention all day and night. But to sustain that level of giving, you must also receive.

This can come in small, everyday ways. Receiving a warm meal. Receiving a hug or an encouraging text. Receiving support from a lactation consultant, a therapist, or a doula. Receiving spiritual or community connection, if that speaks to you. It may also mean *reclaiming pleasure* in your life: listening to music, drinking your favorite tea, or taking a walk in nature.

When you allow yourself to receive, you refill your cup and send a powerful message to yourself: I am worthy of care, too.

Remember: Your Baby Benefits When You Care for Yourself

Sometimes self-care is easier to justify when we realize how deeply it supports our babies, too. A regulated, rested, emotionally attuned parent helps create a calm and secure attachment. Your well-being is the soil from which your child's growth blooms.

When you model healthy boundaries, rest, emotional expression, and self-love, you are also shaping the environment your baby learns from. They don't need a perfect parent. They need a parent who is present and human, a parent who makes room for joy, healing, and self-compassion.

No One-Size-Fits-All Approach

Every family's journey is unique. What works for one may not work for another. Some parents have more hands-on support, while others are navigating it alone. Some are healing from traumatic births, while others are adjusting to parenting multiple children. The key is to **trust your instincts** and **ask for what you need,** even when it's hard.

Self-care doesn't always look the same every day. It will evolve as your baby grows and as your needs shift. What matters is that you keep coming back to yourself with tenderness and intention.

Closing Thoughts: A Gentle Reframe

Balancing caregiving with self-care is not a luxury. It's a foundation. When you tend to your needs, you are not taking time *away* from your baby, you are pouring energy *into* your ability to show up with love, patience, and presence.

By integrating these holistic practices of accepting help, releasing expectations, making space for yourself, you create a nurturing rhythm that supports not just your baby's development but your transformation as well.

Beyond recovering, you are *Becoming*. And that becoming deserves to be honored, protected, and celebrated.

NATURE IMMERSION

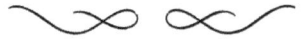

STEP FOUR – ENGAGE

*Definition 1) Occupy, attract or involve
(someone's interest or attention)
2) Participate or become involved in*

In the beginning, your world will revolve entirely around your baby, their schedule, their feedings, their care, and wellbeing. But as the weeks and months pass, you'll gradually find space to let others in and reconnect with the hobbies and activities that brought you joy before motherhood.

It's easy to let your own interests slip away. With so much to do, sitting down to write, draw, or read can feel impossible. But here's the truth...it's not just important, it's essential. When you abandon the things that ground you, you lose more than just a hobby, you lose a piece of yourself. And when that happens, it becomes harder to pass down creativity, joy, and a sense of identity to your children.

Engaging in what makes you *you* strengthens your sense of self and individuality. It also helps establish healthy boundaries early on. Babies are born completely dependent, without a sense of autonomy from their mother. Over time, they learn to self-soothe and develop independence, but they need to see it modeled. When you take time to read, solve a crossword, go for a hike, or join a sip-and-paint night, you're teaching your child (and your partner) something invaluable: Your needs matter. You deserve fulfillment. You are your own person.

Walking Nature Reflection and Activity

Try extending your walk a little longer as you work through this section. You might explore a new route or venture into a different area. As you walk, take notice of how nature preserves itself—how trees, plants, and flowers not only sustain their growth but also instinctively provide for us. Then, observe the wildlife. Notice how their survival is driven by fierce independence, even as they nurture and protect their young. Reflect on these contrasting instincts - nurturing interdependence versus self-sufficiency - and consider how they mirror different aspects of your journey.

LIIT Exercise: Rows with Light Weights

Hold a two-, three-, or five-pound weight in each hand. Stand with your feet shoulder-width apart, arms extended slightly away from your body at your sides. Bend one arm, bringing the weight up toward your chin, then slowly lower it back down. Repeat on the other side. Aim for ten reps on each side. As your strength increases, you can add more repetitions or repeat the exercise two to three times a day.

Mindfulness Breath Practice: 4-4-6 Technique

This simple yet effective breathing exercise helps reduce stress, improve focus, and promote relaxation. Inhale deeply for a count of four. Hold your breath for four seconds. Then exhale slowly for a count of six. Repeat this cycle for one minute. Then allow your breath to return to its natural rhythm, breathing calmly for another five minutes.

Alternative

You can do the walking reflection while walking or jogging in place. If mobility is an issue, try putting on a nature soundscape or a nature scene video with a soft instrumental background.

To modify the exercise, sit upright in a chair to perform the weighted rows. Sitting in a chair helps relieve back tension and provides a sturdy foundation for movement. For an even simpler modification, you can perform the rows without weights, just flex and tense your muscles as you go through the motion.

Dietary Focus: Fun with Salads

Salads are a powerhouse of nutrition, making them an excellent choice during the postpartum period and beyond. Packed with fiber, vitamins, and essential minerals, they support digestion, promote gut health, and help maintain steady energy levels. Leafy greens, such as spinach and kale, provide much-needed iron, while ingredients like nuts, seeds, and avocado offer healthy fats that support hormone balance and brain function. Including a variety of colorful vegetables ensures a broad spectrum of antioxidants, helping the body recover and combat postpartum fatigue. Plus, salads are versatile, easy to prepare, and can be customized to suit your cravings and nutritional needs.

Journal Questions

Another part of the documentation around food is investigating how you are feeling physically. What you eat can affect your mood and energy levels in the long run. *How is my energy level today? Do I feel depleted or balanced? Did I get a chance to eat a full meal?*

During your walk, what parts of nature struck you as self-preserving? What parts showed its nurturing care?

How can you strike a balance between independence and caregiving?

Expression Through Art ~ The Path You Walk

Sketch, paint, or assemble a collage inspired by your walk. Focus on the different paths nature takes, twisting roots, flowing rivers, or winding animal trails. How does this relate to your own path in life?

SECTION V

Finding Joy in the Postpartum Period

CHAPTER 15

NATURE IMMERSION FOR POSTPARTUM HEALING

I hope you have enjoyed the nature immersion activities at the end of each section. Here we dive into why Nature Immersion is so important for healing and recovery. I am a firm believer in Nature Immersion, so much so that this is my second book focusing on Nature Immersion—this time with the postpartum mom in mind. I make it a point to get outdoors daily. Intentionally going outdoors to walk, hike, work in my garden, and to ground.

A Brief History

Forest Bathing, or shinrin-yoku, is a Japanese practice that has been observed for centuries. The practice involves going into a forest and using all of your senses to engage with the environment around you. This is proven to reduce stress, anxiety, improve sleep, and help with weight maintenance. It also helps to boost your mood and immune system. And during postpartum recovery, we need all the mood and immunity boosting we can get!

Modern Times

More recently, many doctors in countries such as Canada, the UK, and the USA are prescribing time outdoors in natural settings to help improve treatment success. In some studies, cancer patients show a higher success rate with treatment when they also integrate walks in the woods. Dr. Millie Roy (Ontario Regional Chair of the Canadian Association of Physicians for the Environment) states, "From increased brain size with improved memory and attention in kids, to improved blood pressure and diabetes in adults, to seniors who live longer and healthier, science is showing that regular time spent in nature achieves all this and more."[11]

Overall health is improved by spending time outdoors. Simple activities like taking a walk, gardening, or sitting in a park can lead to physical and mental improvement.

Benefits for the Postpartum Parent

Engaging with nature is healing on a physical, mental, and spiritual level. It can be tailored to your accessibility and comfort. It's a low-impact way to introduce exercise back into your daily routine and can be shared with family members, including baby.

Spending time outdoors can significantly enhance your mood and overall well-being. Engaging with nature offers a peaceful retreat from daily stressors and fosters a sense of tranquility. Activities such as gentle stroller walks in the park, gardening, or simply relaxing under a tree can provide therapeutic benefits.

How Does Nature Immersion Work?

When in the woods or wooded area, there are organic compounds in the air that we breathe in. These are called VOCs (volatile organic compounds). According to the peer-reviewed research paper, Forest Volatile Organic Compounds and Their Effects on Human Health: A State-of-the-Art Review, "Inhaling forest VOCs like limonene and pinene can result in useful antioxidant and anti-inflammatory effects on the airways, and the pharmacological activity of some terpenes absorbed through inhalation may be also beneficial to promote brain functions by decreasing mental fatigue, inducing relaxation, and improving cognitive performance and mood."[12]

So the saying, "There's something in the air," is not cliché, it is a fact. The composition of trees, the volume of undergrowth, the time of year, and the weather can affect the quantity and quality of these VOCs. Some of these compounds include phytoncides, pinene, and limonene.

The article goes on to mention that the study found, in addition to the benefits of VOCS, the overall (or global) stimulation of the senses and the corresponding areas of the brain further help the physiological and psychological benefits, with vision and eye tracking being the driving factor.

In my opinion, the biggest benefit is that there are no side effects.

My Approach

I chose the name Nature Immersion to honor the notion that Forest Bathing is a traditional Japanese practice. And because I am not Japanese and my culture is very different from the traditional culture, I cannot truly practice Forest Bathing. I can, however, apply the concept to my understanding, and so Nature Immersion was born. Or rather, it's what I choose to call it. In my approach, I combine nature immersion, exercise, self-care, and mindfulness techniques to get a well-rounded experience and a chance to use all my senses in a meaningful way while outdoors.

Quick Ideas for a daily routine:

> Stroller walk
>
> Meditate on the lawn
>
> Journal in a quiet spot in a park or your backyard
>
> Walk holding baby and point out different natural beings such as trees, squirrels, stones, etc.

CHAPTER 16

EMBRACING IMPERFECTION: LETTING GO OF "PERFECT PARENTING"

The pressure to meet unrealistic parenting standards can be overwhelming. It's important to acknowledge that perfection is unattainable and that making mistakes is a natural part of the parenting journey. Practicing self-compassion allows you to release guilt and embrace the learning process. Remember, being a "good enough" parent is more than sufficient for your child's healthy development.

Guilt is a gift that keeps giving, as the saying goes. As a parent and mother, you can lean into feeling guilty about all the things you could have done better. One mother of twins confided in me that she felt guilty to the point of depression when one of the babies ended up with a bad diaper rash. "It's totally my fault. I did not get to them in time, and I was so tired I napped instead of changing them right away."

I assured her that diaper rash was common and even if she managed to change every diaper right away, the baby could still get it. Here is a mother of twin infants, tired, trying her best, and she feels guilty for something that is completely out of her hands. If we let ourselves—if you let yourself—you can come up with a hundred things you'd perceived to have done wrong.

There are going to be days when you will be tired, grumpy, short-tempered. You will have days when you are not focused. There are days when you will make frozen pizzas for the older children, or like me, decide this night is cereal-for-dinner night because you just cannot make another meal. You will have days when you are just not at your best. This is natural and normal for everyone.*

Instead, try focusing on all the hundreds of things you do right. You woke up and got out of bed. You changed a diaper or three. You fed the baby. You washed some dishes. You made a meal. You sat outside for a bit.

You are imperfect, and that's okay. You will make mistakes, but you will do more right than wrong. Learning to forgive yourself for missteps will be important not only for you but also as a trait to pass down to your child. She will learn that she is imperfect, and that's okay. The easier it is for you to embrace yourself, *all of you*, the faster you can move past mistakes and release guilt.

Will you be able to live completely guilt-free? Probably not, but mostly guilt-free is good enough! You are learning with every new phase and stage. You are perfectly imperfect!

Gratitude Practices to Foster Positivity

One way to begin shifting your focus away from guilt and regret is to practice gratitude. Cultivating gratitude can shift your focus from daily challenges to the positive aspects of your life, enhancing your overall sense of happiness and well-being.

One simple yet powerful way to practice this is by keeping a gratitude journal. Take a few moments each day to write down things that bring you joy—no matter how small. Over time, these entries can serve as a reminder of the good in your life, especially on harder days. Reflecting on them regularly helps reinforce a more optimistic and balanced outlook.

You can also build a habit of expressing gratitude in the moment. Practice saying "thank you" out loud or silently whenever something makes you smile or catches your attention. For example, if your favorite song comes on the radio, say, "Thank you." If your baby does something adorable that makes you laugh, whisper a quiet, "Thank you." Even noticing the color of someone's car and appreciating its beauty can be a reason to give thanks. These small, intentional moments of gratitude help train your mind to notice the good, creating a subtle but powerful shift in how you experience daily life.

Gratitude doesn't have to come from big events and in fact, it often grows strongest through simple, everyday moments. Whether it's the warmth of a cup of tea, a kind text from a friend, or a peaceful moment with your baby, acknowledging these experiences helps build emotional resilience. The more you practice, the more naturally gratitude will rise, supporting a more grounded and joyful perspective in your postpartum journey and beyond.

*See earlier chapter about when to seek professional help if these "off" days seem to persist. It is never wrong to call your doctor for help when you are feeling out of sorts.

CHAPTER 17

FUN, SIMPLE ACTIVITIES TO ENJOY WITH YOUR BABY

Engaging in enjoyable activities with your baby strengthens your bond and adds joy to your daily routine. Simple actions such as singing lullabies, dancing around the living room, or creating art together can be delightful for both of you. These shared experiences not only promote your baby's development but also bring lightheartedness to your day.

By incorporating these holistic practices into your postpartum journey, you can create a nurturing environment that celebrates joy and fosters a positive experience for both you and your baby.

Baby Picnic

Bring a soft blanket and head to a shaded area in a park. Let the baby lie down or do tummy time on the blanket while you relax and enjoy a snack. Bring a few favorite toys or books for gentle play.

Library Baby Time or Story Hour

Many libraries offer free infant storytimes with songs, finger plays, and gentle movement. It's great for socializing with other parents and stimulating the baby's senses with music and rhythm. You can get a group together and then go for lunch afterward.

Indoor Mall Walk

Ideal in hot or rainy weather, walk laps in a climate-controlled environment. Stop and look at colorful displays, fountains, or mirrors. Some malls have play areas or family lounges with changing and feeding stations. I like to go early before the shops open, grab a coffee or tea, and walk around the mall to get my steps in. The large displays and aesthetically pleasing colors should be engaging for your little one.

Hiking

Of course, this is my favorite, so we will spend some time here. Hiking can also be challenging with an infant, so making sure you are prepared is important.

Hiking is a great workout and way to connect with nature. If you're used to exploring the outdoors on your own, you may find it challenging to begin hiking again once the baby comes along. You can enjoy the outdoors and even hiking with a baby, toddlers, and teens. The key is to be prepared.

When can I take the baby on her first hike?

This is dependent on several factors. The first of which is: How do you feel? It is recommended that, other than light walking exercise, you wait until six to eight weeks postpartum. This is for vaginal birth with little to no complications. If you've had a C-section, you may want to wait a little longer to account for any stitches and healing that needs to take place.

The second thing to take into consideration is, of course, your baby. At four weeks or less, your baby has little to no motor control. Their muscles are not strong enough to handle the possible jostling a hike could cause. Another key factor is your baby's inability to regulate their temperature. So she can get overheated or very cold quickly. So, it is best to wait until at least four weeks, and recommendations are (like mom) to wait at least six to eight weeks before taking the baby out on a hike. Instead, you can opt for a walk on a flat paved surface with your infant in a stroller.

What gear should I bring?

When you are both ready to step away from the paved paths and hike the trails, there are a few **baby-centric hiking accessories** you may want to try:

- Formula or breast milk in a bottle
- Wipes
- Diapers
- Sun hat
- Light/Heavy jacket

For You:

- Water
- Electrolytes
- Snacks

This list will vary with the time of year you are hiking. Bring a bag to pack out (*pack out* is a hiking term used to describe making sure not to leave anything behind, like garbage or dirty items) soiled clothing and diapers. You may also want to carry a diaper rash cream and a thin changing pad to place on top of your jacket for diaper changes.

Baby Carriers

There are several kinds of carriers for a variety of price points. Just make sure that when using a carrier, he can hold his head upright. The kind of carrier you buy will depend on the type of hiking you are doing. Is this a short one- to two-mile hike? Or will you venture out on a longer trail? Will there be shady areas, or is the trail in the sun? Are you solo hiking with your little one, or will you be with a partner or group?

On a shorter hike, you can use a smaller, lighter weight carrier. While on a longer hike of two miles or more, you may want to opt for a larger back carrier that can double as your backpack. When hiking in a group or with a partner, you can take turns carrying baby.

How long can we stay out?

When deciding how long to stay out on your hike, you will want to take into account the baby's age, the weather, and your stamina. As mentioned before, an infant younger than three months cannot regulate his body temperature, so staying out too long can be detrimental to his health. If you are carrying your baby, pay attention to your body. Are you getting tired? The walk out might have been great, but remember, if it's not a loop, the hike back out can be more treacherous, as being tired can cause you to misstep, putting you and he at risk for a fall. This is especially true if you have a pack full of diapers, bottles, wipes, changes of clothing, and water for yourself. This added weight will cause you to fatigue sooner. Take breaks often and hydrate to keep up your energy.

What should my baby wear?

We touched on this a little bit in an earlier section. Here is a little more detail.

Dress her in layers. Long sleeves are best to provide protection from the sun in the summer and cold and wind in winter. Layers are recommended so that you can remove sweaters or jackets but still have adequate clothing.

Sun hat. This will help keep the sun off her face and reduce the risk of sunburn.

Baby sunglasses. Yes, they make sunglasses for babies. He will look stylish, and this will protect his eyes from UV rays and glare.

Blanket. A blanket may be a good way to provide extra warmth in the cooler months and can be positioned to allow for ventilation so he does not overheat.

Rain Gear and again Rain Gear. Even if it is sunny and there is less than a 0 percent chance of rain, always carry rain gear. I have been on so many hikes when it rained out of nowhere. While a sun shower may be okay, even refreshing, a downpour or rain on a cold day will be at best uncomfortable and at worst a threat to wellbeing.

Hiking is a great way to introduce wellness and a love of nature to your infant right from the start. Begin slowly by taking easy paved paths, and then as your baby gets a little older, venture out on short trails. Bring plenty of water and supplies to keep your baby happy and comfortable. Take breaks often. Remember, it's the experience, not the distance, when it comes to hiking with your baby!

NATURE IMMERSION

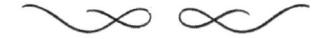

STEP FIVE - SOLITUDE

*Definition 1) The state or situation of being alone.
2) A lonely or uninhabited place.*

I won't downplay this—finding time for solitude in the early weeks and months after your baby's birth will be challenging. But it's also necessary. You need space to think, to plan, to organize your thoughts, or to simply sit and exist without anyone needing something from you.

Solitude is where you can express your needs and desires without fear of judgment. It's where you can reflect on your actions and choices, making space for growth. Even just five minutes a day can make a difference. Prioritize yourself.

Time alone isn't selfish. It's essential. Solitude and silence can increase self-awareness, reduce stress, provide emotional clarity, and improve decision-making by strengthening the prefrontal cortex function. But let's be clear, solitude is not the same as isolation. In solitude, you reconnect and refresh so you can be fully present. Isolation, on the other hand, is about withdrawal and can signal deeper emotional needs that may require support.

Right now, you don't need to escape. You just need to give yourself a little space and time.

Walking Nature Reflection and Activity

During your walk, find a tree that stands taller or is larger than the rest. Observe the space around it—how its branches stretch wide and high, how its roots extend and anchor deep into the earth. Notice its position in relation to the surrounding trees. Reflect on what has allowed this tree to grow taller and stronger. Even though it stands apart, it remains connected, sharing resources, offering shelter, and receiving nourishment in return. Consider how this balance of strength and connection mirrors your own journey.

LIIT Exercise: Overhead Lifts

This is another weighted exercise. Choose a weight of two, three, or five pounds. Stand with your feet shoulder-width apart and bend your arms until your fists are level with your chin. Press the weight overhead slowly, counting to ten, then lower and repeat on the other side. If you're able, complete two sets of ten reps per side.

Mindfulness Breath Practice: Diaphragmatic Breathing

Lie on your back with your knees bent. Place one hand over your heart and the other on your belly. Breathe slowly and deeply, feeling the rise and fall beneath your hands. Continue for as long as you like.

Diaphragmatic breathing offers numerous benefits. It strengthens your diaphragm, reduces strain on your lungs, and conserves energy by slowing your breath. It can also help regulate your metabolism and curb cravings by helping you emotionally regulate, making it easier to lessen emotional eating. Most importantly, in this moment, it provides you with the solitude needed to slow down, reconnect, and decompress.

Alternative

In your favorite nature reflection spot, march or jog in place while observing or visualizing a houseplant. To keep it strong and thriving, you trim away dying leaves and nurture new growth by transplanting new shoots to new pots, giving it space to flourish on its own. In the same way, you must create time for solitude—prune distractions and allow yourself room to grow.

To modify the exercise, skip the weights. Focus on engaging your muscles by tensing or flexing as you move. Start with one set of ten reps per side.

Dietary Focus: Teas and Warm Drinks

Sipping warm herbal teas in the postpartum phase offers both physical and emotional nourishment. Herbal blends like chamomile, nettle, red raspberry leaf, and fennel can support healing, boost hydration, and promote relaxation. Warm drinks provide comfort, help to ease stress, support digestion, and encourage milk production for breastfeeding mothers. Beyond their physical benefits, the ritual of preparing and enjoying a soothing tea fosters moments of mindfulness and self-care, which are essential for postpartum recovery and well-being.

Journal Reflections

Is there anything you wish you had more support with (meal prep, reminders to eat, etc.)? Did you get a chance to eat a meal alone today? How does that make you feel?

As you spend time in solitude, reflect on how you feel in these moments. Do you experience peace, or do worries arise? What does your body and mind need to feel truly at ease with being alone?

Consider how practicing solitude has influenced you. Has it changed the way you interact with your baby, older children, partner, or other family members? Take a moment to explore these thoughts and write about your experience.

Expression Through Art ~ Echoes of Solitude

Using your journal reflections as inspiration, create a visual representation of your ideal experience of solitude. This could be a painting, drawing, collage, or mixed media piece that captures the emotions, environment, and essence of what solitude means to you. Consider incorporating elements that evoke peace, reflection, and self-connection—whether it's a quiet forest, an open sky, a cozy corner, or an abstract expression of stillness.

SECTION VI

Honoring Fathers and Partners on the Postpartum Path

Patresence

The postpartum journey is not one that belongs to the mother alone—it's a transformation for the entire family. As a postpartum doula, I've witnessed the quiet strength, the loving worry, and the deep devotion of fathers and partners. Often, their stories go untold, their emotions tucked behind a brave face as they strive to "be strong" for everyone else. But they, too, deserve to be supported, seen, and nurtured in this tender season of life.

"We're both healing, adjusting, and learning how to be a family."

It's easy to focus solely on the baby and birthing parent—and rightly so, given the physical and emotional demands of childbirth. But partners are also navigating new identities, roles, and responsibilities. They may feel unsure, disconnected, or even helpless in the face of sleep deprivation and emotional highs and lows. In this section, we will delve into the role fathers play, how they can be supportive, how they can get support, and ideas on maintaining a strong relationship in this time of change.

Let this chapter be a gentle invitation to fathers and partners: your presence matters more than perfection. You do not need to fix everything. You're, instead, invited to walk alongside your partner in this journey.

CHAPTER 18

THE INVISIBLE STRUGGLE: FATHERHOOD AND MENTAL HEALTH AFTER BIRTH

"I could see she was in so much pain, and there was nothing I could do about it. I have never felt more helpless in my life."

"I wanted to be there as a father, but I couldn't."

"I really don't know what to do with any of this stuff, so I let her handle it."

These are just a few of the honest, raw statements I've heard from fathers in the postpartum period. Their pain, confusion, and quiet suffering often remain invisible in the larger narrative surrounding birth and parenting. While the focus rightfully stays on the birthing parent's recovery and emotional wellbeing, fathers and non-birthing partners frequently wrestle with their own transitions—often silently.

The Quiet Shift

Non-birthing partners and fathers can have varied emotional and psychological responses to pregnancy and the postpartum period. For some, there is deep awe and love in witnessing their child's birth. For others, there may be a growing sense of fear—fear of not being enough, fear of harming the baby, or fear of failing their partner.

Many fathers report a loss of intimacy, a diminished libido, or feeling emotionally sidelined. Some experience jealousy—not of the baby—but of the closeness between mother and child. Others grieve the loss of their old relationship dynamic, freedom, or even the person they were before parenthood.

Often, they don't speak up about these emotions. Society still teaches men that they must "be strong," "tough it out," and "be the rock" for their families. Instead of opening up, they quietly carry the burden of confusion, shame, or helplessness. They suppress their fears because they feel that expressing them would be selfish or disrespectful when their partner is physically recovering from childbirth.

When Connection Feels Like Isolation

Some fathers feel an intense emotional bond with their baby and partner right away. They might take on more responsibilities at home, step away from social circles, or even take extended time off work. But in doing so, they can begin to feel the same kind of isolation that many mothers report. The difference is few people are asking how *they're* doing.

Many fathers find themselves in a strange limbo. They're expected to be providers, supporters, and protectors but rarely are they given the space or tools to process their own emotions or shifts in identity. The transition to fatherhood is profound, but culturally, we've minimized it.

Paternal Postpartum Depression and Anxiety

Yes, fathers can experience postpartum depression and anxiety too. It's estimated that **one in ten fathers** develops symptoms of paternal postpartum depression (PPPD), and that number increases significantly if their partner is also struggling with a perinatal mood disorder.

The symptoms may look different in fathers than in mothers. Instead of sadness and crying, their depression may show up as:

- Irritability or frequent anger
- Emotional numbness or detachment
- Increased alcohol or substance use
- Withdrawing from family and friends
- Loss of interest in hobbies or relationships
- Feeling overwhelmed, hopeless, or trapped
- Changes in appetite or sleep patterns
- Feeling unappreciated, invisible, or like they're failing

They may not even recognize what they're experiencing as depression or anxiety. They may just feel like they're failing at something they were "supposed" to be naturally good at.

Why Support for Fathers Matters

Supporting fathers is not just about helping *them*. Doing so supports the entire family unit. A mentally healthy father is better able to bond with his baby, support his partner, and adapt to the ongoing changes of parenthood.

Here's what can help:

- **Therapy:** Talking to a licensed professional can provide a safe space to work through emotions and reframe negative thought patterns.
- **Peer Support Groups:** Whether online or in person, these spaces can normalize fathers' experiences and reduce shame.
- **Honest Conversations:** Talking with other dads, friends, or supportive family members can reduce the feeling of isolation.
- **Co-Parenting Education:** Learning about baby care and infant development together with a partner can foster connection and shared responsibility.
- **Check-ins with Providers:** Just like moms are screened at postpartum visits, fathers can also benefit from emotional wellness check-ins during pediatric appointments or family therapy sessions.

You Deserve Support, Too

If you are a father or non-birthing partner reading this, please know your feelings are valid. Your mental health matters. You deserve space to grieve, to grow, to learn, and to be cared for. You deserve to not be okay sometimes and you deserve support in finding your way back to wholeness.

We cannot continue to build strong families without making room for the emotional lives of *all* parents.

CHAPTER 19

SHOWING UP WITH LOVE: EVERYDAY WAYS TO SUPPORT AND STAY CONNECTED

The postpartum period is a time of enormous change—for everyone. While the birthing parent is healing and adapting, the non-birthing partner is also transforming. There is no script for how to do it perfectly. But presence, empathy, and small, thoughtful gestures go further than perfection ever could.

1. Be Present, Not Perfect

You don't need to have all the answers. You don't need to "fix" everything. Presence is often the most powerful support you can offer.

- Holding the baby so the birthing parent can shower in peace
- Prepping a simple meal or snack before they even have to ask
- Sitting beside them during a quiet moment of overwhelm—no advice, just your company

These small acts are not insignificant. They are the threads that weave safety, trust, and emotional closeness in the fabric of early parenthood. Your steady presence sends the message: *You're not alone.*

> *Reminder: Listening without judgment is one of the most healing gifts you can give.*

2. Ask, Don't Assume

Even with the best intentions, assumptions can create distance or resentment. Instead of guessing what your partner needs, ask her.

Try asking questions like:

> "What would help you feel cared for right now?"
>
> "Would it help if I took the baby for a walk so you can rest?"
>
> "Do you need a nap, a snack, a stretch, or a quiet moment?"
>
> "Is there anything that's felt hard today that you want to talk about?"

These open-ended, caring questions show your willingness to support without controlling. They also open up space for honesty and deeper connection.

> *Tip: Let your partner's answer guide your actions and be ready for the needs to change from hour to hour.*

3. Learn and Grow Together

Parenting is not about already knowing what to do—it's about learning together, one messy day at a time.

- Read about newborn development, postpartum recovery, and mental health together
- Watch parenting videos or attend classes as a team
- Ask questions at pediatrician appointments or lactation consults—be engaged

When you show that you're *in it together*, it reinforces your bond and encourages shared responsibility. The baby belongs to both of you. So does the learning curve.

> *Shared learning fosters mutual respect and eases the mental load on the birthing parent.*

Keeping the Relationship Nourished

The romantic relationship often takes a back seat in the whirlwind of newborn care—but love doesn't disappear just because you're exhausted. In fact, this season is when love needs *intentional tending*.

Nurture Each Other Through Micro-Moments

Small gestures make a big difference:

- A gentle kiss on the forehead while passing by
- A lingering hug in the kitchen, even with the baby crying
- A whispered "I love you" when the lights go out

These micro-moments remind each other that *I still see you. I still choose you.*

Celebrate Each Other

Parenting can feel like an endless loop of tasks. It's easy to feel unseen. Make it a point to name and notice each other's efforts:

- "You're doing such a great job with the baby."
- "I noticed you got up three times last night. Thank you."
- "I appreciate how patient you were today."

Words of affirmation are not fluff—they are fuel.

Gratitude keeps the heart open, even when the body is running on empty.

Communicate Gently

Tensions will rise. Misunderstandings will happen. But how you talk to each other can either deepen your bond or build walls.

- Use "I feel" statements instead of accusations: "I feel overwhelmed when the baby cries and I don't know how to help."
- Create space for check-ins: "How are *you* feeling about everything lately?"
- Listen to understand, not just to reply.

Pause arguments when you're both too depleted. Come back when you're calmer. Compassion first. Always.

Final Thought: The Gift of Showing Up

There is no perfect parent and no perfect partner. Being present, being willing, and being kind are all that truly matter. The baby may not remember every bottle or every lullaby but they will feel the love that filled the room. And so will your partner.

Your support, your curiosity, your efforts to grow together. These are not small things. They are everything.

A Note from Ghene't

As someone who has walked this journey with families time and time again, I want to say to all partners:

> You are an anchor.
>
> Your care, your listening, your sleepless nights, and your silent sacrifices are felt. Even if not always spoken aloud your support and presence are appreciated.
>
> Thank you for showing up.

For all my mother's, first-timers and beyond:

Embracing joy during the postpartum period is essential for both your well-being and your baby's development. Integrating holistic practices can help you discover moments of happiness and fulfillment amidst the challenges of new motherhood. You are doing great, and even on the days when you only feel at 50 percent, you are always 100!

NATURE IMMERSION

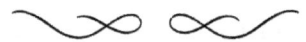

STEP SIX - I AM

*Definitions I 1) Singular pronoun, myself AM
1) First person singular of be. Used to bring a person
or thing into the present. The Latin root word
of AM is LOVE*

Recently, my daughter and I were talking about college, new friends, and what I used to do at her age. I told her how proud I was that she's focused—not distracted like I was, going to clubs and parties. She gasped, "Wait! You went to a club?"

I laughed, "Yeah."

She stared at me. "My mom went to a club? I can't believe it! What else are you hiding?"

I smiled and said, "Well, I wrote three fantasy novels. Never published them, but I did write them."

She looked at me, wide-eyed, then responded, "Oh my gosh! I don't even know you!"

We both laughed.

She is nineteen years old, and by the time you're reading this, probably twenty. For nineteen years of her life, she only knew one version of me. And that's okay.

But what's not okay is for me to forget all the versions of myself.

One of the things that largely goes unspoken is the sense of self a mother has after having a baby. Some women lose their sense of identity. It can feel like every moment of every day is commanded by children—diaper changes, potty training, schoolwork (if you have older kids). Breakfast, lunch, dinner, cleaning, and making time for your partner. And that's without even considering the demands of returning to work.

Somewhere in the midst of all this, we begin to disappear.

While having children changes you forever, the I AM practice allows you to begin reimagining who you are—to remember who you were and decide who you want to be. Begin to think in terms of I AM.

I AM a mother.

I AM a woman.

I AM a chef.

I AM a designer.

You are more than just one thing. And although that one job—motherhood—is the most important you will ever do, you are still more.

If you were an artist, you are still an artist.

If you were a writer, you are still a writer.

If you were a doctor, you are still a doctor.

You are all those things and so much more.

Having a child can dramatically change the way we see ourselves. We can get lost. We can feel invisible. We are constantly serving, and who we are on the inside becomes hidden, small.

You have every right to hold on to who you are—even if you currently present only one version.

Walking Nature Reflection and Activity

Spend a little longer walking during this practice. If you can, set a goal to reach thirty minutes. Responsibilities call to all of us, and even if you can't always make it to the full thirty, simply setting the goal will help you stay out longer.

Throughout this Nature Immersion practice, you've observed the trees, the birds, the wind. You've felt the warmth of the sun and maybe even the cool kiss of rain. You've watched chipmunks and squirrels at play and may have even wandered into new areas, parks, or trails. These moments have moved you, deepening your connection to the world around you—and to yourself.

Now, take a moment to observe one of these things more closely. SEE beyond what's in front of you. That squirrel isn't just a squirrel. She may be a mother, a sister, a child. She gathers food, cracks open a nut, and as the hull falls to the earth, it decomposes—nourishing the forest floor. The trees stand tall, rooted in their purpose, steadfast and sure.

So as you walk, look beyond the surface. See the deeper story in everything around you.

LIIT Exercise: Sit and Stand

Sometimes, the most effective exercises are the simplest. This movement helps strengthen your core, improve mobility, and support knee health. And believe me, your knees are important!

Find a sturdy chair or even use your couch. Simply sit, then stand. Try to do it without using your hands. It's similar to a squat, but with the added support of the seat beneath you, making it easier on your knees. To get the most out of it, engage your core as you move. Small movements like this can make a big difference!

Mindfulness Breath Practice: 4-7-8 Method

Breathe in for four seconds, hold for seven seconds, then exhale slowly for eight seconds. This simple yet powerful breathing technique helps regulate your breath, bringing a sense of calm and control. By slowing your breathing, you can reduce stress, one of the biggest triggers for food cravings. Since stress hormones often drive those cravings, using this method may help you pause, reset, and make more mindful choices.

Alternative

Do the above walking nature reflection as you jog or walk in place. You may decide that yoga or stretching may be better on some days. Listen to your body. Stretching and yoga are great for joint lubrication, flexibility, and toning muscles. The sitting and standing exercise might be a bit challenging if you had a C-section or a complicated birth, so take it easy. Feel free to use your hands for support, and try sitting on a chair instead of a couch—it's firmer and higher, making it easier to stand up from. Listen to your body and go at your own pace!

Dietary Focus - Snacking Alternatives

Swapping out unhealthy snacks for nutritious alternatives can be both beneficial and enjoyable! Healthier options like fresh fruit, nuts, yogurt, or air-popped popcorn can satisfy cravings while providing essential nutrients. Experimenting with different flavors and textures (crunchy veggie chips or protein-packed energy bites) can make the switch feel exciting rather than restrictive. Plus, choosing smarter snacks helps maintain energy levels, supports overall health, and encourages mindful eating habits.

Journal Questions

What are you grateful for in your body today? What's one way you can be more intuitive about eating? Has your relationship with food changed at all since you started journaling? In what ways?

What did you observe in nature today? Did you look beyond its surface? Reflect on what you saw and any deeper insights it revealed to you.

Expression Through Art ~ I Am Me

Create a visual representation of yourself in any way that feels right to you. It could be a drawing, an abstract piece, a collage, or even a collection of items you've gathered on a walk. Use this as a form of self-expression. How do you see yourself? Let your creativity guide you.

BONUS JOURNAL REFLECTION

Review the definitions from the previous steps. Did any of them surprise you? How did they make you feel? Take a moment to reflect and write about your thoughts, impressions, and how these meanings connect to your own experiences.

Nature Immersion for Postpartum Healing

NATURE AS YOUR GUIDE: WALKING INTO YOUR NEXT SEASON

Your journey to improved well-being doesn't end here. Postpartum recovery is just one season of your life, and as the years go by, there will be moments of growth, challenge, and transformation. Caring for yourself (body, mind, and spirit) will always require intention, but you don't have to do it alone.

One beautiful way to continue your healing is through nature. Whether it's a quiet solo walk to reconnect with yourself or a family hike to strengthen bonds, time spent outdoors can be a powerful tool for recovery, reflection, and renewal. I would love to continue supporting you on this path. Stay connected with me for more guidance, encouragement, and resources, including healing hikes designed for postpartum recovery and family connection.

As a thank-you for being here, I have a special free gift just for you!

Email ghenetleeyong@gmail.com with subject Nature Immersion for Postpartum Healing

Follow my socials below for ongoing free support on your journey. You deserve this time for yourself.

Website and Blog - familyholisticpracticespostpartumdoulaservicewithghenetlee-y.com
Instagram - instagram.com/family_holistic_ppdoula
YouTube - @PostpartumCarewithGhenet

With love and encouragement,
Ghene`t Lee-Yong

ACKNOWLEDGMENTS

I want to give the warmest of thanks to Elicia, my dear friend, who has helped with reading and proofreading in the early stages of writing this. Her insights and questions helped hone my message and clarify details. I thank Ruby for fact-checking and always reading with her eyes open. I also want to thank publisher and writing coach extraordinaire Shanda Trofe and her team, including my editor, Shelby Rawson, for their guidance and support in editing, advice, and help getting this book out into the world.

It can be a tricky thing to get thoughts on to page in a way that makes sense and is cohesive. They made that possible.

I thank my children. Their patience and encouragement have meant the world to me. They are my motivation and strength. They are my muse to keep writing, creating, and designing.

I also want to acknowledge the many friends and professionals who helped me fact-check so that I could bring trustworthy holistic practices to you.

And of course, I thank all of you, my readers, for trusting me with your time. I truly hope you are able to find peace and recovery through Nature Immersion.

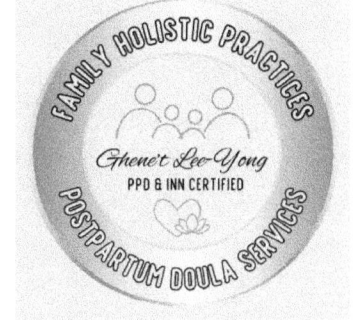

APPENDIX I

RECIPES

Section One: Soups
Healthy Homemade Ramen (Serves 4-6)

Ingredients:

4 cups mixed vegetables of your choice (e.g., carrots, sweet peppers, bok choy)

2 cups protein of choice (leftover stewed chicken recommended)

1 large onion, diced

4 cloves garlic, minced

1 tsp ginger (fresh or powdered)

2 tbsp coconut aminos or soy sauce (gluten-free and "no soy" options available)

Salt, to taste

Pepper, to taste

Adobo seasoning, to taste

½ tsp red pepper flakes (optional)

2 cups water

4 cups chicken or vegetable broth (Adjust if using leftover stewed chicken. You may need to use less or more. See instructions below.)

8 oz udon rice noodles

Instructions:

1. Prepare the Protein

If using fresh meat, stew it with half of the diced onion, half of the garlic, and 2 cups of water.

Add salt, pepper, adobo seasoning, and just a dash of ginger.

Let it simmer until fully cooked.

If using leftover stewed chicken, set aside and reserve the broth.

2. Prepare the Vegetables

While the meat is cooking, dice the vegetables, onion, and garlic.

In a sauté pan, cook the remaining onion and garlic until slightly browned.

Add vegetables and a light layer of seasoning (excluding ginger).

Cook until the vegetables reach your preferred texture, then reduce heat to low.

3. Combine & Simmer

Once the meat is fully cooked, transfer it to the sautéed vegetables. Reserve the stew water.

Drizzle with soy sauce or coconut aminos and mix well.

Transfer everything to a soup pot and add the reserved stew water.

Pour in up to 1 cup of water and 4 cups of broth.

Season with additional soy sauce or coconut aminos, a dash of ginger, and red pepper flakes (if using).

Let the soup simmer on low heat for 10–15 minutes, stirring occasionally.

4. Cook the Noodles & Serve

While the soup simmers, cook the udon rice noodles according to package instructions.

To serve, place the cooked noodles in bowls and ladle the soup over the top.

Quick Tip

For a faster version, use leftover stewed meat and simply add water, soy sauce, or coconut aminos, and seasoning to taste before pouring over cooked noodles.

Enjoy this nourishing and flavorful soup, perfect for a cozy meal!

Section Two: Stews
Dairy-Free, Gluten-Free Hearty Chicken Stew (Serves 4-6)

Ingredients:

1 ½ lbs boneless, skinless chicken thighs or breasts, cut into bite-sized pieces

2 tbsp olive oil or coconut oil

1 large onion, diced

3 cloves garlic, minced

3 carrots, sliced

2 celery stalks, chopped

1 medium sweet potato or Yukon gold potato, diced

1 red bell pepper, chopped

1 zucchini, chopped (optional)

4 cups chicken broth (gluten-free)

1 cup full-fat coconut milk (for creaminess)

1 tsp turmeric

1 tsp dried thyme

1 tsp smoked paprika

½ tsp ground cumin

1 bay leaf

Salt and pepper, to taste

1 cup frozen peas (optional)

2 tbsp fresh parsley, chopped (for garnish)

Juice of ½ lemon (for brightness)

Instructions:

1. Sauté the Base

In a large pot or Dutch oven, heat the oil over medium heat.

Add the diced onion and garlic, sauté until fragrant (about 2 minutes).

Add the chicken pieces, season with salt and pepper, and cook until lightly browned (5 minutes).

2. Add Vegetables & Spices

Stir in the carrots, celery, sweet potato, bell pepper, and zucchini (if using).

Add the turmeric, thyme, smoked paprika, cumin, and bay leaf. Stir to coat everything in the spices.

3. Simmer the Stew

Pour in the chicken broth and bring to a gentle boil. Reduce heat, cover, and let simmer for 20–25 minutes until the vegetables are tender.

Stir in the coconut milk and frozen peas (if using). Let simmer for another 5 minutes.

4. Final Touches & Serve

Remove the bay leaf. Stir in fresh parsley and squeeze in the lemon juice for added brightness.

Taste and adjust seasoning as needed.

Serve warm as is or with cauliflower rice or gluten-free bread on the side.

Enjoy this comforting, creamy, and nourishing stew!

Section Three: Fruit, Yogurt, and Oatmeal
Creamy Dairy-Free Fruit & Yogurt Bowl (Serves 2-3)

Ingredients:

2 cups dairy-free yogurt (coconut, almond, or cashew-based)

1 cup mixed fresh fruit (e.g., strawberries, blueberries, mango, banana, or kiwi)

2 tbsp chia seeds or flaxseeds (for added fiber and omega-3s)

¼ cup granola (gluten-free if needed)

1 tbsp shredded coconut (optional)

1 tbsp honey or maple syrup (optional, for extra sweetness)

1 tsp vanilla extract (optional, for flavor)

½ tsp cinnamon (optional)

Instructions:

1. Prepare the Base

In a bowl, mix the dairy-free yogurt with vanilla extract and cinnamon (if using).

2. Assemble the Bowl

Divide the yogurt into serving bowls.

Top with fresh fruit, spreading it evenly over the yogurt.

3. Add Texture & Flavor

Sprinkle with chia seeds or flaxseeds for extra nutrients.

Add granola for crunch and shredded coconut for a tropical touch.

Drizzle with honey or maple syrup if you prefer a sweeter taste.

Enjoy!

Serve immediately or refrigerate for 10-15 minutes to let the flavors blend.

This fruit and yogurt bowl makes a delicious breakfast, snack, or light dessert!

Simple & Creamy Oatmeal Recipe (Serves 2)

Ingredients:

1 cup rolled oats (gluten-free if needed)

2 cups water or dairy-free milk (almond, coconut, or oat milk)

1 tbsp maple syrup or honey (optional)

½ tsp cinnamon (optional)

½ tsp vanilla extract (optional)

1 pinch of salt

Toppings (Optional):

Fresh fruit (bananas, berries, apples)

Nuts or seeds (almonds, walnuts, chia, flaxseeds)

Nut butter (peanut, almond, or cashew)

Shredded coconut

Instructions:

1. Cook the Oats

In a saucepan, bring the water or dairy-free milk to a boil.

Stir in the oats and a pinch of salt.

2. Simmer & Stir

Reduce heat to low and let simmer for about 5 minutes, stirring occasionally, until the oats are soft and creamy.

3. Add Flavor

Stir in maple syrup or honey, cinnamon, and vanilla extract for extra taste.

4. Serve & Top

Pour into bowls and add your favorite toppings. Enjoy!

Serve warm and enjoy a cozy, nourishing meal!

Section Four: Fun with Salads
Savory & Sweet Super Salad with Goat Cheese (Serves 4-6)

Ingredients:

6 cups mixed greens (spinach, arugula, or your choice)

1 cup fresh berries (strawberries, blueberries, or raspberries)

2 medium beets

1 bell pepper (any color), sliced

½ small red onion, thinly sliced

2 cloves garlic, minced

1 cup shredded carrots

½ cup crumbled goat cheese

Instructions:

1. Roast the Beets.

Preheat your oven to 400°F.

Scrub and dry the beets, then cut them into wedges or dice them. Season if desired.

2. Lightly grease a baking pan with coconut oil or butter.

Arrange the beets in a single layer and roast for 20-30 minutes, until tender.

Once done, let them cool for about 5 minutes before peeling.

3. Prepare the Salad:

While the beets are roasting, chop the vegetables and combine them with your greens in a large bowl.

4. Assemble & Serve:

Add the roasted beets to the salad.

Top with goat cheese and fresh berries.

For added protein, you can include your choice of meat (such as grilled chicken or salmon).

Make It Easier:

Roast the beets ahead of time and store them in the refrigerator or freezer for quick meal prep.

Enjoy this nutrient-packed, flavorful salad that perfectly balances savory and sweet!

Section Five: Teas and Warm Drinks

You can find teas in a number of places, in your local grocery, in a farm market store, or you can order online.

Calming Chamomile & Lavender Tea (Great for relaxation and postpartum recovery)

Ingredients:

1 tbsp dried chamomile flowers

1 tsp dried lavender buds

1 tsp honey or maple syrup (optional)

1 cup hot water (just below boiling, about 190°F)

1 slice of lemon (optional)

Instructions:

1. Add chamomile and lavender to a tea infuser or teapot.

2. Pour hot water over the herbs and let steep for 5–7 minutes.

3. Strain and sweeten with honey or maple syrup if desired.

4. Add a slice of lemon for a refreshing twist.

Sip and relax!

Spiced Ginger & Turmeric Tea (Anti-inflammatory and warming)

Ingredients:

1-inch piece fresh ginger, sliced (or 1 tsp dried ginger)

½ tsp ground turmeric (or 1-inch fresh turmeric root, sliced)

1 cinnamon stick (or ½ tsp ground cinnamon)

1 cup hot water

½ tsp honey or maple syrup (optional)

½ tsp lemon juice (optional)

Instructions:

1. Add ginger, turmeric, and cinnamon to a small pot with 1 cup of water.

2. Simmer on low heat for 10 minutes to infuse the flavors.

3. Strain the tea into a mug.

4. Stir in honey or maple syrup for sweetness and add lemon juice for brightness.

Enjoy the warm, spicy goodness!

Section Six: Snack Alternatives

For Sweet Cravings

- Fresh Fruit with Nut Butter – Apple slices or bananas with almond or peanut butter
- Frozen Grapes or Berries – Naturally sweet and refreshing.
- Dark Chocolate (70% or higher cacao) – A small piece satisfies chocolate cravings without excessive sugar.
- Chia Pudding – Mix chia seeds with coconut milk and a dash of honey or maple syrup, then refrigerate overnight.
- Baked Apples or Pears – Sprinkle with cinnamon and bake for a warm, sweet treat.
- Homemade Energy Bites – Blend dates, nuts, cocoa powder, and coconut for a natural, no-bake snack.
- Greek or Coconut Yogurt with Honey & Berries – A creamy, protein-rich alternative to ice cream.

For Salty Cravings

- Roasted Chickpeas – Crunchy, salty, and packed with protein.
- Air-Popped Popcorn with Nutritional Yeast – A healthy swap for buttered popcorn with a cheesy, savory taste.
- Homemade Kale Chips – Toss kale with olive oil and sea salt, then bake until crispy.
- Nuts & Seeds – Lightly salted almonds, cashews, or sunflower seeds make for a satisfying crunch.
- Avocado Toast on Gluten-Free Crackers or Bread – Sprinkle with sea salt and chili flakes for a flavorful bite.

- Cucumber Slices with Hummus – A fresh and hydrating option.
- Olives or Pickles – Naturally salty and full of gut-friendly probiotics.

Nut-Free
For Sweet Cravings
- Fresh fruit (berries, apple slices, grapes, bananas, mango, etc.)
- Fruit kabobs (a fun mix of melon, pineapple, strawberries)
- Applesauce (unsweetened or cinnamon-spiced)
- Dried fruit (raisins, apricots, mango—just check for no added sugar or sulfites)
- Frozen grapes or banana slices

Crunchy & Sweet
- Graham crackers
- Nut-free granola (made with seeds, oats, and dried fruit)
- Rice cakes with honey or seed butter
- Cereal snack mix (using nut-free cereals like Cheerios, Chex, etc.)
- Kettle corn or caramel popcorn

Creamy & Cool
- Yogurt with fruit or granola (Greek, coconut-based, or regular)
- Chia pudding with vanilla or cocoa
- Frozen yogurt tubes or nut-free ice pops
- Pudding cups (chocolate or vanilla)

Baked & Packaged Treats
- Oatmeal raisin cookies (nut-free recipe or store-bought)
- Fig bars (like Nature's Bakery – check label for nut-free status)
- Mini muffins (banana, blueberry, etc.)
- Marshmallows or nut-free rice crispy treats

Crunchy & Savory
- Popcorn (air-popped or lightly salted; try flavors like sea salt, olive oil, or kettle corn)
- Pretzels (classic twists, sticks, or pretzel crisps—check for nut-free brands)
- Roasted chickpeas (seasoned with garlic, paprika, or sea salt)
- Seaweed snacks (crispy, salty, and light)
- Cheese crackers (like Cheez-Its or Annie's Cheddar Bunnies)
- Tortilla chips with salsa or guacamole
- Pita chips with hummus

Protein-Packed
- String cheese or cheese cubes
- Hard-boiled eggs with a dash of salt
- Turkey or beef jerky (look for nut-free labels)
- Deli meat roll-ups (with cheese or pickles inside)

Fresh & Crisp
- Cucumber slices with salt and vinegar
- Pickles or olives
- Cherry tomatoes with a sprinkle of sea salt
- Celery sticks with cream cheese or sunbutter (if safe)

BIBLIOGRAPHY

1. March of Dimes. "Postpartum Depression." *March of Dimes*. Accessed August 15, 2025. https://www.marchofdimes.org/find-support/topics/postpartum/postpartum-depression.

2. American Psychological Association. "Advancing Social Connection as a Public Health Priority in the United States." *American Psychological Association*. Accessed August 15, 2025. https://www.apa.org/search?query=social%20connection.

3. Kühn, Simone, Ulrike Schmidt, Sandra H. Wittfeld, and Jürgen Gallinat. "A One-Hour Walk in Nature Reduces Amygdala Activity in Women, but Not in Men." *Frontiers in Psychology* 13 (2022): 931905. https://www.frontiersin.org/journals/psychology/articles/10.3389/fpsyg.2022.931905/full.

4. Harvard Health Publishing. "Pregnancy's Lasting Toll." *Harvard Health*. Updated October 1, 2022. https://www.health.harvard.edu/womens-health/pregnancys-lasting-toll.

5. Ke, F., and N. W. Newton. "The Powerful Impact of Music." *Intersect: The Stanford Journal of Science, Technology, and Society* 12, no. 2 (2019). https://ojs.stanford.edu/ojs/index.php/intersect/article/view/2873.

6. Bechard-Laroche, Annie. "Affirmations May Improve Life Satisfaction and Well-Being." *Psychology Today*, July 21, 2023.

https://www.psychologytoday.com/us/blog/the-age-of-overindulgence/202307/affirmations-may-improve-life-satisfaction-and-well-being.

7. Fallon, V., R. Groves, H. Halford, and R. Harrold. "Associations between Postpartum Depression and Assistance with Household Tasks and Childcare during the COVID-19 Pandemic: Evidence from American Mothers." *BMC Pregnancy and Childbirth* 21 (2021): 593. https://bmcpregnancychildbirth.biomedcentral.com/articles/10.1186/s12884-021-04300-8.

8. Smyth, Joshua M., Melissa M. Nazarian, and Megan M. Hockemeyer. "Online Positive Affect Journaling in the Improvement of Mental Distress and Well-Being in General Medical Patients with Elevated Anxiety Symptoms: A Preliminary Randomized Controlled Trial." *JMIR Mental Health* 5, no. 1 (2018): e6305886. https://pmc.ncbi.nlm.nih.gov/articles/PMC6305886/.

9. Wong, Jessica, and Tatia M. C. Lee. "Maternal Postnatal Confinement Practices and Postpartum Depression in Chinese Populations: A Systematic Review." *Frontiers in Global Women's Health* 4 (2023): 1061530. https://pmc.ncbi.nlm.nih.gov/articles/PMC10615300/.

10. Holt, Luther Emmett. *The Care and Feeding of Children.* New York: D. Appleton and Company, 1894.

11. Living Architecture Monitor. "Nature Prescriptions: The Growing Trend of Doctors Prescribing Time Outdoors." *Living Architecture Monitor*, Fall 2024. https://livingarchitecturemonitor.com/articles/growing-trend-of-doctors-prescribing-time-outdoors-fa24.

12. Calfapietra, Carlo, Paola Fares, Giorgio Manes, and Alessandra Loreto. "Forest Volatile Organic Compounds and Their Effects on Human Health: A State-of-the-Art Review." *International Journal of Environmental Research and Public Health* 20, no. 3 (2023): 1815. https://doi.org/10.3390/ijerph20031815.

ABOUT THE AUTHOR

Ghene`t discovered the doula profession as a young mother, and after years of working in early childhood education and supporting families through every stage, she finally found her true calling. She specializes in overnight care, offering gentle newborn support, feeding assistance, and emotional reassurance to ensure both baby and parents feel nurtured. Whether you need a full night's rest or guidance through nighttime feedings, she creates a calm, supportive environment tailored to your family's needs.

One of her favorite things to hear from parents is, *"I fell asleep and woke up, and it was morning!"* Her passion is making sure moms, birthing parents, partners, and families get what they need most during this time. **Rest.**

"I love helping families during this sacred transition. My work with children and families has shown me how vital emotional health is for the mother, baby, and entire family. Everyone needs time, siblings need one-on-one moments with their parents, babies need round-the-clock care, moms need rest and recovery, and parents need time to connect with each other."

Ghene`t strives to be a calm, peaceful, and non-intrusive presence, relieving tension and providing space for families to navigate this delicate transition.

When she's not supporting families, you can find her hiking, spending time with her children, and writing.

HOW TO GET MORE HELP

One-on-One Support

I offer Virtual Postpartum Services tailored to your needs. If you're looking for personalized guidance and support, please follow the link or scan the QR code to visit my website for more details.

I look forward to being a part of your journey and providing the support you deserve!

bit.ly/41wCek1

Join My Community

Are you seeking a safe and welcoming space to connect with other mothers? Look no further! Join my private support group on Skool, **Wildflowers: Postpartum & Beyond,** where you can share your experiences, ask questions, and uplift one another in your parenting journey. Whether you're navigating the early stages of motherhood or balancing the challenges of raising older children, you'll find understanding, encouragement, and friendship here.

Come be a part of a non-judgmental community that celebrates all stages of parenting. We can't wait to welcome you!

www.skool.com/wildflowers-im-growing-too-4146

www.ingramcontent.com/pod-product-compliance
Lightning Source LLC
Chambersburg PA
CBHW070620030426
42337CB00020B/3860